Understanding
Thyroid Disorders

Dr Anthony Toft

Published by Family Doctor Publications Limited
in association with the British Medical Association

IMPORTANT

This book is intended not as a substitute for personal medical advice but as a supplement to that advice for the patient who wishes to understand more about his or her condition.

Before taking any form of treatment
YOU SHOULD ALWAYS CONSULT YOUR MEDICAL PRACTITIONER.

In particular (without limit) you should note that advances in medical science occur rapidly and some information about drugs and treatment contained in this booklet may very soon be out of date.

Family Doctor Publications, PO Box 4664, Poole, Dorset BH15 1NN

ISBN-13: 978 1 903474 19 8
ISBN-10: 1 903474 19 1

19952013

Contents

About the author

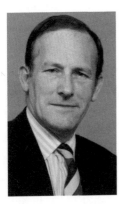

Dr Anthony Toft CBE, LVO, MD, FRCP was, until recently, a Consultant Physician and Endocrinologist at the Royal Infirmary of Edinburgh where he specialised in the diagnosis and treatment of patients with thyroid disease. He has published numerous articles in the leading medical journals in the world. Dr Toft has been President of the British Thyroid Association, President of the Royal College of Physicians of Edinburgh, and a Physician to Her Majesty the Queen in Scotland. He is now in private medical practice in Edinburgh.

Introduction

What is the thyroid gland?

The thyroid gland lies in the front of the neck between the skin and the voice box. It has a right and left lobe each about five centimetres in length and joined in the midline. The entire gland weighs less than an ounce (about 20 grams). Despite its small size it is an extremely important organ which controls our metabolism and is responsible for the normal working of every cell in the body.

Thyroid hormones

The thyroid gland achieves this control by manufacturing the hormones (see Glossary, page 102) thyroxine (T_4) and triiodothyronine (T_3) and secreting them into the bloodstream.

Iodine is an important constituent of these hormones. There are four atoms of iodine in each molecule of thyroxine, hence the abbreviation T_4, and three atoms of iodine in each molecule of triiodothyronine or T_3.

Doctors believe that T_4 starts to be active only when it is converted, mainly in the liver, to T_3 by the removal

Iodine-deficiency goitre

The red areas on this world map show the regions of the world in which iodine-deficiency goitre is a common disorder. This occurs largely as the soil, and consequently food, lacks sufficient iodine.

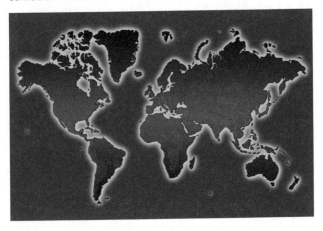

of one atom of iodine. In parts of the world where there is a severe lack of iodine in the diet, such as the Himalayas, there is not enough iodine for the thyroid gland to make adequate amounts of T_3 and T_4. In an attempt to compensate, the thyroid gland enlarges to form what is known as a goitre, which is visible. If this extra manufacturing capacity is still inadequate, the patient develops an underactive thyroid gland (see page 38).

Iodine deficiency is not present in the UK. Sometimes too much iodine in the diet causes the thyroid gland to produce excessive amounts of thyroid hormones. This can also be a result of medication.

Thyroid gland

The thyroid gland lies in the neck between the skin and the voice box (larynx). The thyroid gland is a butterfly-shaped gland consisting of two lobes, one on each side of the trachea (windpipe).

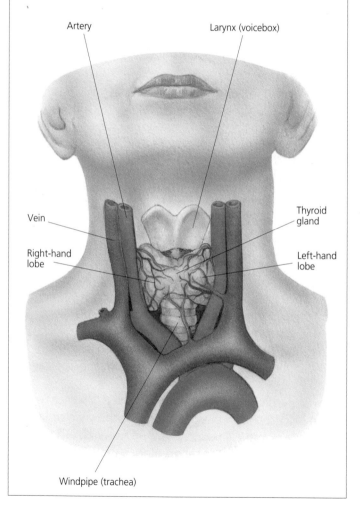

Artery

Larynx (voicebox)

Vein

Thyroid gland

Right-hand lobe

Left-hand lobe

Windpipe (trachea)

Balancing the hormones

In healthy people the amounts of T_3 and T_4 in the blood are maintained within narrow limits by a hormone known as thyroid-stimulating hormone (TSH) or thyrotrophin. TSH is secreted by the anterior pituitary gland which is a pea-size structure, hanging from the undersurface of the brain just behind the eyes, and enclosed in a bony depression in the base of the skull.

When thyroid disease causes thyroid hormone levels in the blood to fall, TSH secretion from the pituitary is increased; when thyroid hormone levels rise, TSH secretion is switched off – a relationship known as 'negative feedback', familiar to engineers and biologists.

Thyroid hormone production

The production of thyroid hormones by the thyroid gland is regulated by the pituitary gland, which produces thyroid-stimulating hormone (TSH) in response to the levels of thyroid hormones in the blood.

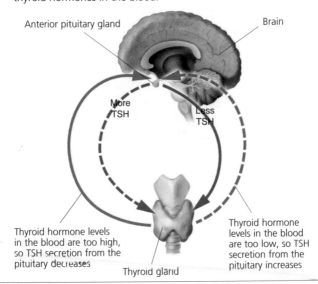

Anterior pituitary gland

Brain

More TSH

Less TSH

Thyroid hormone levels in the blood are too high, so TSH secretion from the pituitary decreases

Thyroid hormone levels in the blood are too low, so TSH secretion from the pituitary increases

Thyroid gland

Hypothyroidism and hyperthyroidism

If your GP suspects that you may have an underactive thyroid gland (hypothyroidism), his or her diagnosis can be confirmed by sending a sample of your blood to the laboratory for analysis. Low levels of T_3 and T_4 and high levels of TSH in your blood mean that your doctor was right. Similarly, the diagnosis of an overactive thyroid gland (hyperthyroidism) is confirmed by high levels of T_3 and T_4 and low levels of TSH. The results will be available within a few days.

Patients with uncomplicated hypothyroidism will not usually be referred to hospital and your GP can prescribe and monitor your treatment. Most patients with hyperthyroidism or with abnormal growth of the thyroid gland will be referred to a hospital specialist for further investigation and advice about treatment.

Thyroid disease is common and hyperthyroidism, hypothyroidism or abnormal growth or enlargement of the gland (goitre or thyroid nodule) affects about one in 20 people. Most diseases of the thyroid can be successfully treated, and even thyroid cancer, which is rare, may not lead to a reduction in life expectancy if detected early and treated appropriately.

Thyroid disease often runs in families but in an unpredictable manner, and certain forms are associated with an increased risk of developing conditions such as diabetes mellitus or pernicious anaemia. All types of thyroid disease are more common in women.

The following chapters deal with each of the most common thyroid disorders individually.

Case history

Ahmed was born in a village in the high mountains of northern Pakistan where he spent most of his childhood.

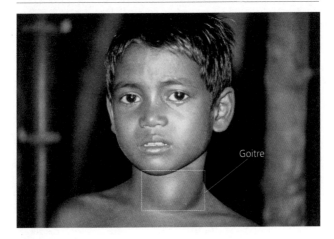

Goitre

At the age of 20 he came to London to study engineering when, at a routine medical examination, he was noticed to have a goitre. He felt well and all the thyroid tests were normal.

The cause of the goitre was attributed to iodine deficiency when Ahmed told the doctor that most of the people in his village also had a goitre. His diet had contained enough iodine to prevent the development of hypothyroidism, but his goitre is likely to remain, even though he has decided to live the rest of his life in a part of the world where there is an adequate amount of iodine in his diet.

KEY POINTS

■ Thyroid disease is common, affecting around one in 20 people

■ More women than men are affected

■ Your GP can diagnose the condition with a simple blood test

■ Treatment is usually successful, and even thyroid cancer can be cured if caught early

Overactive thyroid

Graves' disease

An overactive thyroid gland (hyperthyroidism or thyrotoxicosis) results from the over-production of the thyroid hormones, thyroxine or T_4 and triiodothyronine or T_3, by the thyroid gland. In three-quarters of patients this is the result of the presence in the blood of an antibody (see Glossary, page 102) that stimulates the thyroid, not only to secrete excessive amounts of thyroid hormones but also, in some, to increase the size of the thyroid gland, producing a goitre.

This type of hyperthyroidism is known as Graves' disease, named after one of the physicians who described the condition in considerable detail over 200 years ago.

The cause of the antibody production is not known but, as Graves' disease runs in families, genes (see Glossary, page 102) must play a part. There is thought to be some environmental trigger that starts off the disease in genetically susceptible individuals, but the culprit, unless it is an iodine-containing drug, such as amiodarone used in the treatment of heart disease,

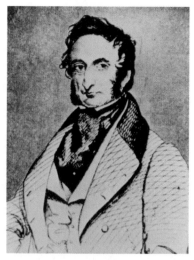

Robert Graves, 1796–1853

is difficult to identify. Stress, in the form of major life events, such as divorce or death of a close relative, may play a role.

Some patients with Graves' disease develop prominent eyes (exophthalmos or proptosis) and a few also suffer from raised, red, itchy areas of skin on the front of the lower legs or on the top of the feet, which are known as pretibial myxoedema. These, like the production of the thyroid-stimulating antibodies, are caused by an abnormality in the patient's immune system which doctors don't yet fully understand. Most other patients with hyperthyroidism have a goitre containing one or more nodules or 'lumps'. These over-produce thyroid hormones in their own right and are not under the control of TSH, as is the normal thyroid gland.

Graves' disease can come on at any age but most commonly affects women aged 40 to 50 years. About a third of all patients will have a single episode of hyperthyroidism lasting several months. The rest will have successive episodes of hyperthyroidism over many years. Unfortunately, it is not possible to predict the pattern of hyperthyroidism when it first occurs. Hyperthyroidism resulting from a nodular goitre is unusual before the age of 40 and, unlike in some patients with Graves' disease, it persists indefinitely once it has developed.

What is the pattern of development?

In retrospect, most patients will have had symptoms for at least six months before they go to see their doctors, but in some, usually teenagers, the onset is more rapid with symptoms present for only a few weeks. Not all patients with hyperthyroidism have all the symptoms listed below. In elderly people the predominant features, in addition to weight loss, are often a reduction in appetite, muscle weakness and apathy. A young woman, on the other hand, may appear to be full of energy and be unable to sit still for more than a few seconds.

Symptoms of an overactive thyroid
Weight loss
This happens to almost all patients as a result of a 'burning off' of calories caused by the high levels of thyroid hormones in the blood. You will probably find you're hungry all the time, and that you even have to get up in the night to get something to eat. The degree of weight loss varies from 2–3 kilograms to as much as 35 kilograms or more, but a few people find that their appetite increases to such an extent that they may gain a little weight. If you are severely overweight when the condition first starts, you'll probably be delighted

How the hyperthyroidism of Graves' disease behaves over time

This chart shows the course of the hyperthyroidism of Graves' disease if it is left untreated.

About a third of patients (group A) would have an isolated episode of overactivity, lasting several months followed by prolonged remission and eventually, after 10 to 20 years, by the onset in some of an underactive thyroid.

In the majority of patients (group B) there will be frequent remissions followed by relapses.

An 18-month course of an antithyroid drug, such as carbimazole (see page 18), would probably be successful in patients in group A, but recurrent hyperthyroidism would probably develop in patients in group B, usually within 2 years of stopping the drug.

It is not possible to decide with any accuracy which group you belong to at your first presentation with Graves' disease.

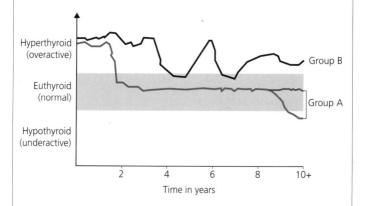

Group A = represents approximately one-third of patients with untreated hyperthyroidism

Group B = represents approximately two-thirds of patients with untreated hyperthyroidism

to find that you're losing weight and put it down to dieting, but sadly you'll put the weight back on once you're being treated.

Heat intolerance and sweating

As metabolism is increased, your body produces excessive heat which it then gets rid of by sweating. You won't enjoy warm weather or a centrally heated environment and may feel comfortable scantily dressed on a crisp winter's day. In extreme cases, your inability to tolerate heat may lead to disagreements with friends and colleagues as you're constantly turning heating thermostats down, opening windows and tossing blankets or duvet off the bed.

Irritability

This most often affects women with a young family. You may find yourself increasingly unable to cope with the demands and stresses of looking after the children, lose your temper frequently, and find that you're abnormally sensitive to criticism, bursting into tears for no apparent reason. You may find it difficult to concentrate, which can adversely affect your performance at school, college or work.

Sleep disturbance and altered energy levels

Hyperthyroidism acts on the brain in a way that is similar to an overdose of caffeine, initially creating a feeling of extra energy. With mild hyperthyroidism, this may be felt as a benefit initially, but quickly gives way to disturbed sleep, an inescapable feeling of useless energy and a sensation of being unable to rest or even sit still.

It often results in worsening fatigue or even exhaustion, partly because of sleep deprivation. This in turn worsens the irritability, emotional instability and lack of concentration, which also come from hyperthyroidism.

Palpitations

Most patients experience palpitations (rapid or fluttering heart beat), or you may be aware of your heart beating at a faster rate than normal. In severe, long-standing, untreated hyperthyroidism, particularly in elderly people, there may be an irregular heartbeat, known as atrial fibrillation, and even heart failure.

Breathlessness

This is most likely to be noticeable when you've exerted yourself, for example, after climbing two or three short flights of stairs. Individuals with asthma may notice a worsening of their symptoms.

Tremor

Most patients complain of shaky hands which may be mistaken by friends and relatives for the tremor of alcoholism. You'll find it difficult to hold a cup still or insert a key into a lock and your handwriting may deteriorate.

Muscle weakness

Characteristically, the thigh muscles become weak, making it hard to climb stairs or to get up from a squatting position or a low chair without using your arms.

Bowel movements

There tends to be an increase in their frequency such that you pass a softer than normal stool two or three times daily. Diarrhoea can occasionally be a problem.

Menstruation

Periods are often irregular, light or even absent. Until the hyperthyroidism is adequately treated it may be difficult to conceive.

Skin, hair and nails

You may find that your whole body itches, and people with Graves' disease, as mentioned earlier, may develop raised itchy patches on their lower legs and feet (pretibial myxoedema). Your hair will probably become thinner and finer than usual and won't take a perm very well. Rarely, patients with Graves' disease may develop patchy areas of baldness known as alopecia areata. This is a separate autoimmune condition affecting the hair follicles, which fluctuates in severity. It is not influenced by treatment of the hyperthyroidism and requires management by a dermatologist.

There may be significant and even dramatic hair loss a few weeks after treatment of your hyperthyroidism as a result of the rapid fall in thyroid hormone levels. You will not become bald and there will be re-growth of a healthy head of hair. Your nails will be brittle and become rather unsightly.

Bone loss and osteoporosis

Hyperthyroidism accelerates the loss of bone that often affects women after the menopause. Untreated, this can lead to an increased risk of fractures.

Eyes

It is only those patients with Graves' disease who have trouble with their eyes. Problems include excessive watering made worse by wind and bright light, pain and grittiness as if there is sand in the eyes, double vision and blurring of vision. Many sufferers are also naturally upset because they develop exophthalmos (protruding eyes) as well as 'bags' under their eyes.

Goitre

Although you will obviously be able to see when you have a goitre, it's unlikely to cause any actual symptoms other than a sensation that there is something in your neck that shouldn't be there.

Confirming the diagnosis
Blood test

You'll probably have had a blood test taken at your health centre or GP's surgery, but you may well have more done for confirmation when you go to the outpatients' clinic at the hospital.

Thyroid scan

The specialist may also wish to carry out a thyroid scan to obtain more information about the cause of the hyperthyroidism as this may affect the type of treatment that you will need.

A thyroid scan requires a tiny dose of radioactive iodine or technetium to be given either by mouth or by injection into a vein. The dose is so small that it can even be given to someone who is known to be allergic to iodine. Most specialists, however, would try to avoid radioactive scanning if you are pregnant or breast-feeding.

After your GP has made the initial diagnosis, you'll probably have to wait for a bit before you can see the hospital specialist. In the meantime, your symptoms may be eased by taking one of the beta-blocker drugs such as propranolol, which counteracts to some extent

Blood test

For a blood test a vein is chosen and the injection site cleaned. A hollow needle attached to a syringe is inserted into the vein and blood drawn out for testing.

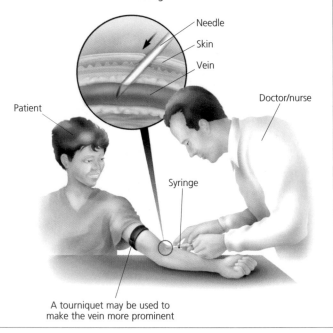

Needle

Skin

Vein

Doctor/nurse

Patient

Syringe

A tourniquet may be used to make the vein more prominent

the actions of thyroid hormones. This is most likely to be in a dose of 40 milligrams to be taken three or four times daily or in the form of propranolol (Inderal LA) 160 milligrams daily as a single dose by mouth. Beta-blocking drugs should not be taken by individuals with asthma.

Treatment for Graves' disease

There are three forms of treatment for the hyperthyroidism caused by Graves' disease. These are drugs, surgery and radioactive iodine.

Thyroid scan

Isotope scanning uses a gamma camera to create a picture from radiation emitted from the body after a radioactive isotope, such as technetium-99m, has been injected.

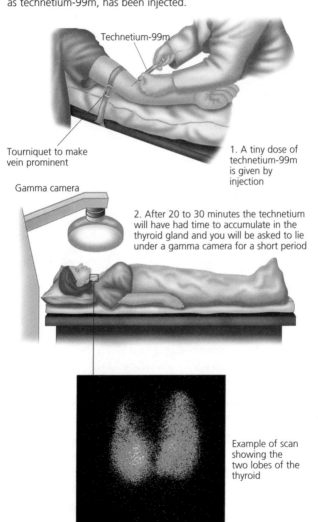

Technetium-99m

Tourniquet to make vein prominent

1. A tiny dose of technetium-99m is given by injection

Gamma camera

2. After 20 to 30 minutes the technetium will have had time to accumulate in the thyroid gland and you will be asked to lie under a gamma camera for a short period

Example of scan showing the two lobes of the thyroid

How antithyroid drugs work

Antithyroid drugs interfere with the manufacture of thyroid hormones, bringing the high levels found in hyperthyroidism back to normal.

Before drug
Thyroid gland is over-producing thyroid hormones

After drug
Thyroid hormone levels restored to normal

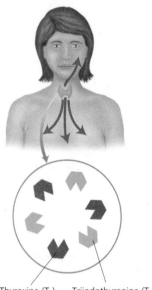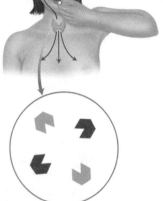

Thyroxine (T$_4$)   Triiodothyronine (T$_3$)

Drugs

Antithyroid drugs are usually given to younger patients who go to their doctor when they have their first episode of hyperthyroidism. The most commonly used drug in the UK is carbimazole which reduces the amount of hormones made by the thyroid gland. It is available as 5 milligram and 20 milligram tablets. A high dose (40 to 45 milligrams daily) is used initially and your symptoms should start to improve after 10 to 14 days, but it will be 4 to 6 weeks or more before you feel back to normal.

Normally treatment is continued for 6 to 18 months, in the hope that you are one of those who will have a single episode of hyperthyroidism. To start with, your specialist will review your treatment every 4 to 6 weeks, and the dose of carbimazole will be reduced in stages down to 5 to 15 milligrams daily in a single dose, depending upon the results of measurements of your blood levels of T_3, T_4 and TSH.

Some specialists prefer to give a high dose of carbimazole throughout treatment, usually as 40 milligrams daily, in the form of two 20 milligram tablets. If this high dose were to continue for several weeks or more, you would eventually develop an underactive thyroid gland and therefore thyroxine is added to the carbimazole once thyroid hormone levels have returned to normal. The advantage of this type of treatment is that it doesn't need to be reviewed so often. It can also be particularly beneficial for patients with severe eye disease, but isn't any more effective in controlling symptoms of hyperthyroidism than carbimazole alone.

What you should know about drugs
Few people will experience any side effects from taking carbimazole, but those who do usually develop them within three to four weeks of starting treatment. A skin rash affects two per cent of patients. It is very itchy, covers the whole body and looks as if you have been stung by a nettle. Doctors call the blisters urticaria. You should stop the carbimazole and inform your doctor. The rash will disappear within a few days and the itch will be helped by antihistamine tablets. The most

serious side effect is a reduction in the number of white blood cells (agranulocytosis) which results in a very sore throat with mouth ulcers and a high fever.

The low white cell count makes you prone to infection with bacteria. Agranulocytosis is a medical emergency and you must contact your doctor immediately and insist on an appointment that day. Fortunately it is rare, developing in one in 300 to 500 patients. Although the white cell count always recovers, you will need to take antibiotics and may even be admitted to hospital for a short period. Most sore throats are the result of run-of-the-mill viral infections, but, even if you think that your sore throat is trivial, you should request a blood count for reassurance. Other side effects include sore joints, slight scalp hair loss and headache.

If you do develop a side effect while taking carbimazole, you can be given an alternative drug called propylthiouracil, which works in the same way. Abnormal liver blood tests may rarely develop, particularly in patients taking high doses of propylthiouracil during the first weeks of treatment. The problem usually disappears when the dose is reduced, although occasionally the drug must be withdrawn. If you smoke, the antithyroid drugs will take longer to be effective and there is a greater chance of the overactive thyroid returning after treatment has stopped.

Surgery

Unfortunately, despite taking carbimazole or propylthiouracil alone or in combination with thyroxine for up to 18 months, more than half of all patients will develop hyperthyroidism again and usually within 2 years of stopping the drug. If you're under 45 when

Surgery

Surgery may be the treatment of choice in a young patient with Graves' disease and a large goitre.

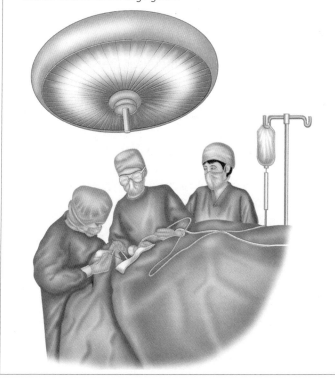

you have your second bout of the condition, it may be treated surgically by removing about three-quarters of your thyroid gland.

Before this operation can be done, however, it is necessary to restore thyroid hormone levels in your blood to normal with carbimazole.

Once you've been given a date for the operation, you may be asked to take an iodine-containing medication for 10 to 14 days before surgery to reduce the size of the thyroid and its blood flow, which makes the job technically simpler for the surgeon. You'll usually go into hospital the day before your operation, which lasts about one hour, and you'll be allowed home two days later.

What you should know about surgery

The disadvantage is that you will have a scar, but this usually becomes pale and unnoticeable among the other wrinkles in the neck. Alternatively you can wear jewellery or scarves to hide it.

In very rare cases (less than one per cent), the parathyroid glands, which lie close to the thyroid and control the level of calcium in the blood, may be damaged, in which case long-term treatment with vitamin D tablets will be necessary.

Equally rare is damage to one of the nerves supplying the voice box which may result in significant alteration to the quality of the voice. Although this wouldn't matter very much to most people, it could make surgery a less acceptable option to anyone who depends upon their voice for a living – an opera singer, for example.

In experienced hands the initial results of surgery are good. Eighty per cent of sufferers will be cured immediately. However, 15 per cent will have had too much thyroid tissue removed and so will be hypothyroid, whereas 5 per cent will have had insufficient thyroid tissue removed and remain hyperthyroid. These failures are not the result of surgical incompetence, but have more to do with the nature of the underlying thyroid disease. What's more, over the passage of time, an increasing proportion of those patients whose hyperthyroidism was originally cured by surgery will develop an underactive thyroid gland. Recurrence of hyperthyroidism may even develop 20 to 40 years after apparently successful surgery. In the event of recurrent hyperthyroidism, it is unusual to consider a second operation because surgery will be technically difficult and the risk of damage to surrounding structures increased. To prevent the possibility of recurrence, some surgeons prefer to remove the entire thyroid gland (total thyroidectomy) with guaranteed hypothyroidism, and the need for life-long dependence on thyroid hormone replacement.

Radioactive iodine (iodine-131)

Traditionally this form of treatment is reserved for patients aged over 40 to 45 and beyond child-bearing age or for younger individuals who have been sterilised.

This conservative approach was originally adopted because of concern that radioactive iodine might lead to any children conceived after treatment being born with abnormalities. In fact, there is no evidence for this, and in some hospitals there is a move towards using radioactive iodine in younger patients as it is cheap and easy to administer.

Radioactive iodine is taken as a capsule or a drink that tastes like water, and is usually administered in hospital in a department of medical physics. Before receiving treatment you will be asked to sign a consent form, and will have received instructions about avoiding places of entertainment and close contact with colleagues and young children for a period of a few days after therapy. With heightened security at airports you may trigger the alarm systems for several weeks after treatment with radioactive iodine. Many clinics will now issue a card indicating that you have

Radioactive iodine treatment

Radioactive iodine is taken up by the thyroid gland, where it destroys part or all of the thyroid tissue, reducing the production of thyroid hormones.

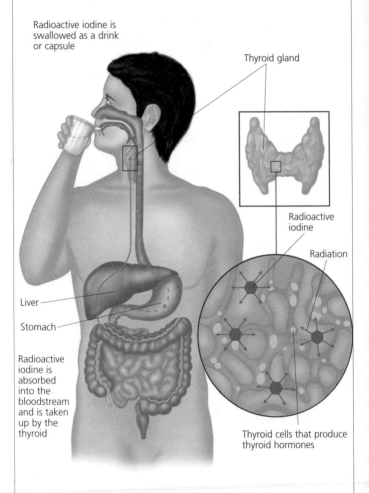

Radioactive iodine is swallowed as a drink or capsule

Thyroid gland

Radioactive iodine

Radiation

Liver

Stomach

Radioactive iodine is absorbed into the bloodstream and is taken up by the thyroid

Thyroid cells that produce thyroid hormones

Choosing which treatment is right for you

- No treatment is perfect and you will need to discuss the options with your specialist. Some patients are not keen on surgery even when a course of antithyroid drugs has been tried and failed.

- There is no reason why you shouldn't have a second or even a third course in the hope that the disease will ultimately 'burn itself out'. Indeed, before there was any form of treatment for the hyperthyroidism of Graves' disease, a proportion of patients got better spontaneously after months or years and then became hypothyroid. Some patients are content to take a small dose of carbimazole for several years after their first relapse rather than experience repeated episodes of hyperthyroidism; this is quite safe.

- Some patients are unhappy at the prospect of radioactive iodine treatment and some specialists consider that the best treatment for a young patient with severe hyperthyroidism and a large goitre is surgery.

- Whatever kind of treatment you have for hyperthyroidism, you will need regular follow-up, usually by an annual blood test taken at a health centre or your GP's surgery.

been treated, which you should carry with your travel documents for the next six months.

Radioactive iodine is never prescribed for pregnant women as it will adversely affect the fetal thyroid gland and women are advised to avoid pregnancy for four months after treatment.

Radioactive iodine acts by destroying some of the thyroid cells and by preventing others from dividing, which is how they are normally replaced at the end of their lifespan. The treatment takes six to eight weeks to work and in the interim, depending upon the severity of the hyperthyroidism, you may be given propranolol or carbimazole to relieve your symptoms. If you had been started on carbimazole beforehand, you will be asked to stop the drug 48 hours before the radioactive iodine treatment. You'll be asked to come back to hospital for a check-up in two to three months and, if you're one of the minority of people who is found to be still hyperthyroid, you'll be given a second dose of radioactive iodine.

What you should know about treatment with radioactive iodine

The major problem with this treatment is, however, the development of hypothyroidism. It's most likely to appear in the first year after treatment, affecting about 50 per cent of people in some centres. In each year after that, around two to four per cent of people will be affected. It follows that the great majority become hypothyroid eventually and it is essential that you should have regular check-ups either at the hospital or with your GP. Once hypothyroidism has developed treatment is with thyroxine, ultimately in a dose of 100 to 150 micrograms daily. There are no side effects with thyroxine if the appropriate dose is taken regularly.

Case history

Although 70-year-old John Parry considered himself to be generally very healthy, he had recently noticed that his ankles were swelling. To start with, it was just at night, but then it happened all the time and his legs felt very heavy.

One night at 1am he woke up gasping for breath and coughing up white frothy spit. His wife called an ambulance, and John was admitted to the local hospital within 20 minutes. The doctor on duty, Dr Mackenzie, correctly diagnosed heart failure as the cause of the fluid accumulation in John's legs and lungs. He also noticed that John's pulse rate was very rapid and irregular and an electrocardiogram showed this to be caused by atrial fibrillation. Mr Parry was given oxygen using a facemask, an injection of a drug called furosemide (Lasix) to get rid of the excess fluid, and digoxin tablets to reduce the speed of his heart beat. As patients with atrial fibrillation are at risk of throwing off blood clots from the heart, resulting in a stroke or a blocked artery in a leg, he was also given tablets called warfarin to thin the blood.

Dr Mackenzie had at one time worked with an eminent endocrinologist and knew that atrial fibrillation could sometimes occur as a complication of an overactive thyroid gland, particularly in older patients.

Mr Parry did indeed have hyperthyroidism which turned out to be caused by Graves' disease and he was treated with radioactive iodine. He was also given the antithyroid drug, carbimazole, for six weeks until the radioactive iodine had time to take effect.

Although to begin with Mr Parry was concerned about the number of tablets he was taking when he left hospital, these had all been stopped within six months as his thyroid gland came under control. Even his heart is now beating regularly and he is as fit as ever. His GP carries out thyroid blood tests regularly to make sure that Mr Parry is not developing an underactive thyroid gland as a result of the radioactive iodine treatment.

Case history

Anna Robinson had had a previous episode of hyperthyroidism caused by Graves' disease in her mid-20s, for which she had been given an 18-month course of carbimazole. At the age of 45, she noticed that she was troubled by the heat, but put this symptom down to the 'change of life'.

However, when she began to lose weight and her hands became shaky, she realised that her thyroid gland was overactive again. At the local hospital the specialist suggested that she should be treated with radioactive iodine. In spite of reassurances and the evidence that this form of treatment was not associated with any risk other than the eventual onset of an underactive thyroid gland, Mrs Robinson was uneasy. She was aware from articles in the newspapers of a possible link between radiation and leukaemia in those living near to nuclear power stations, and she did not like the thought of avoiding her new grand-daughter albeit only for a few days after treatment.

As she was a keen singer in the local church choir, thyroid surgery was felt not to be appropriate because of the possibility of a change in the quality of her voice.

Mrs Robinson was relieved to learn that there was no reason why she could not be treated with carbimazole now or in the future.

Graves' disease and the eyes
What is happening in the eyes?

If the doctor looks hard enough, most patients with Graves' disease have changes to their eyes known as ophthalmopathy or orbitopathy. Both eyes are usually affected, but often one more than the other. It is better to think of the ophthalmopathy as a separate

Graves' disease

Most patients with Graves' disease will have changes to their eyes. Both eyes are usually affected but often one more than the other.

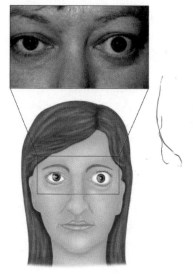

autoimmune condition that frequently coexists with Graves' disease, rather than as a complication of the thyroid disease itself. This helps to explain why eye disease may occur before the onset of the overactive thyroid gland or even for the first time after you have been successfully treated.

There are three phases to the ophthalmopathy: the initial development and worsening, followed by a period of relative stability and then by a variable degree of improvement. Complete disappearance of the eye disease is rare and, even if you feel that your eyes are back to normal, there will be subtle abnormalities evident to a specialist, if not to friends and family.

An early sign is retraction of the upper eyelid which appears as if it has been pulled up, exposing more of the white of the eye and causing a staring appearance. This may improve after the raised levels of thyroid hormone have been restored to normal with treatment. Some patients complain of dry, gritty eyes, as if there is sand in them, and of constant blinking, others of excessive watering.

The other features of thyroid eye disease result from a build-up of pressure behind the eyeball, which sits in a bony socket known as the orbit. The space between the eyeball and the back of the orbit contains the muscles that move the eye, the optic nerve, which relays messages from the retina to the brain, and fat.

In patients with thyroid eye disease, among other changes there is an accumulation of excessive amounts of water behind the eyeball, and the muscles and fat become swollen and boggy. The muscles double or treble in bulk and cease to work efficiently. As a result, the normal movement of the eyes may be restricted and uncomfortable, with double vision (diplopia) and even the development of a squint.

The increase in pressure behind the eyeballs pushes them forwards, producing the 'pop-eye' appearance known as exophthalmos or proptosis. The increased exposure of the protruding eyeballs makes them more prone to irritation from dust, grit, wind and sun, and the cornea may be damaged. In addition, some of the fat behind the eyeballs may be forced into the eyelids, contributing to their puffiness and the appearance of 'bags under the eyes'. Very rarely, in severely affected patients, the increased pressure may damage the optic nerve and cause partial or total loss of vision.

Treatment

Treatment of the eye disease is not as satisfactory as that of the overactive thyroid gland. Smoking is thought to make it worse as does poor control of the hyperthyroidism. It is very important, therefore, that you stop smoking completely and are careful to follow your doctor's instructions about dosage of tablets, such as carbimazole or thyroxine.

Of the three treatments for an overactive thyroid gland, deterioration of the ophthalmopathy is thought to occur most often after radioactive iodine. Some specialists will not wish to prescribe this form of therapy for you if your eyes are badly affected, or they might advise a course of steroids, such as prednisolone

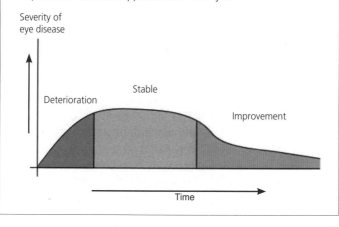

Thyroid-related eye disease: time course of disease

Thyroid-related eye disease usually has three phases, each of variable duration. After an initial deterioration the condition should stabilise over a period of two to three years. Thereafter relatively minor surgery should correct any double vision and improve the cosmetic appearance of the eyes.

Rarer types of hyperthyroidism

- Mild hyperthyroidism, lasting for a few weeks, may occur after a viral infection of the thyroid; this is known as viral or de Quervain's thyroiditis and the most prominent feature is severe pain and tenderness over the thyroid gland associated with symptoms of a flu-like illness. The hyperthyroidism rarely needs any treatment other than a beta-blocking drug, such as propranolol. There usually follows an equally short-lived period of mild hypothyroidism and then full recovery.

- A similar pattern of mild hyperthyroidism, followed by mild hypothyroidism and then recovery, but without pain or signs of a viral illness, occurs three to six months after the birth of a baby in those with underlying autoimmune thyroid disease. This is known as postpartum thyroiditis (see page 104), and as silent thyroiditis when unrelated to pregnancy. It is important to distinguish these types of hyperthyroidism from Graves' disease because they do not require treatment with antithyroid drugs.

- An overactive thyroid may occur for the first time in early pregnancy, when it is usually associated with excessive vomiting or hyperemesis. This is known as gestational thyrotoxicosis. The thyroid is stimulated by a hormone made by the developing placenta, which is similar in make-up to the natural thyroid-stimulating hormone or TSH. The overactivity lasts for a few weeks only and treatment, if necessary, would be with a beta blocker and, only rarely, with carbimazole.

Rarer types of hyperthyroidism (contd)

• The iodine-containing drug, amiodarone, which is used increasingly by heart specialists for the treatment of certain irregularities of heart rhythm, may cause hyperthyroidism. Your blood thyroid hormone levels should be checked before you start taking the drug, and at six-monthly intervals while you're on it.

• Subclinical hyperthyroidism: the combination of a low TSH and normal (usually high normal) T_3 and T_4 in the blood is known as subclinical hyper-thyroidism, because patients have few, if any, symptoms and the abnormality is often detected during a routine health check or because of the presence of a goitre. It is now considered to be the mildest form of thyroid overactivity and treatment may be recommended, even though you are feeling well, in order to prevent the more obvious hyperthyroidism developing in the future, and cancelling out any risk of osteoporosis or even atrial fibrillation.

for six to eight weeks, immediately after the radioactive iodine has been given.

If you have dry eyes, you may find that a prescription for artificial tears helps, as it also does paradoxically for those with excessive watering. It is also worth wearing dark glasses when it is sunny. Double vision may be helped by having prisms fitted to your spectacles.

If you have more advanced eye disease, especially if your vision is deteriorating, you may be treated with prednisolone tablets, often coupled with radiotherapy. This treatment damps down the immune-mediated

Tears in Graves' disease

Tears are produced by the lacrimal (tear) glands. In Graves' disease they may not work as well as normal. If you have dry eyes a prescription for artificial tears may help relieve the discomfort.

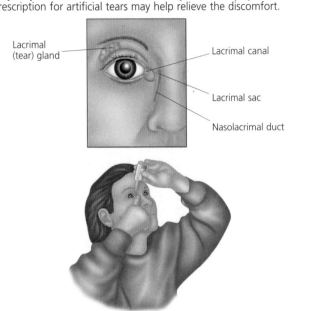

Lacrimal (tear) gland

Lacrimal canal

Lacrimal sac

Nasolacrimal duct

swelling of the tissues behind the eyeball. It is becoming more common to give the steroid (as methylprednisolone) in a course of intravenous injections over several weeks, because this is not only more effective but also causes fewer side effects.

Alternatively, an operation may be required to remove part of the wall of the orbit, thereby reducing the pressure behind the eyeball. Such a major undertaking is rarely necessary, however, and would be carried out only after close collaboration between thyroid and eye specialists.

Most people with Graves' disease find that their eye problems settle down considerably over a period of two to three years. At that stage, relatively minor surgery will correct double vision and reduce the 'staring' look and the bags under the eyes.

Nodular goitre

This is treated either with surgery or with radioactive iodine. Unlike someone with Graves' disease, you're unlikely to develop hypothyroidism.

It used to be fashionable after surgery to prescribe thyroxine to prevent regrowth of the goitre, which is common over a period of some 20 years, but this is not really useful unless you've developed hypothyroidism.

Hyperthyroidism and elderly people

Those in their 70s and 80s or beyond may not have the classic features of an overactive thyroid gland. Although there is usually weight loss, the appetite is often reduced, and the thigh muscles become weak, causing difficulty in climbing stairs, getting out of the bath or rising from a low chair. Instead of being jumpy and fidgety, older patients become apathetic and cannot be bothered doing things. They may be thought, by relatives, to be depressed. Often there is no goitre and there are no eye signs. As a result of this less typical presentation of an overactive thyroid gland, the diagnosis may be delayed, by which time the pulse may be irregular from atrial fibrillation and there may even be heart failure.

Living with someone with an overactive thyroid

It is the irritability, the short fuse and the emotional

rollercoaster that make life difficult for friends and family. No one quite knows what to expect and there is a feeling of walking on eggshells all the time. Mum (and it is usually mum) cannot sit still, and seems to be doing several things at once, although none of them to her usual standard.

Despite being exhausted, she does not sleep and gets up early to do the ironing or clean the house. Nothing pleases her. Trivial incidents, such as breaking a cup or burning the toast, make her 'fly off the handle' or burst into tears.

There is often talk of separation and even divorce as the charged atmosphere in the household over many months takes its toll. If the overactive thyroid develops at the time of the menopause, as it often does, there is frequently delay in diagnosis because the symptoms are inevitably attributed to the change of life. It is only when hormone replacement therapy fails to help that the penny drops.

Once the hyperthyroidism is diagnosed, the family will feel guilty, but tolerance is needed for several weeks or even months after treatment before mum is restored to her old self.

KEY POINTS

■ Around three-quarters of cases of hyper-thyroidism are caused by Graves' disease

■ Many people with Graves' disease may have inherited a tendency to develop it, although other factors are also involved in triggering the condition

■ The people most likely to develop Graves' disease are women between the ages of 40 and 50

■ Drugs, surgery and radioactive iodine are all possible ways of treating Graves' disease, but there is no one treatment that is right for everyone

■ Your specialists may want to discuss the treatment options with you before making the final decision on which approach is best for you

■ After treatment, you will need regular check-ups to ensure that you stay well

■ Most people with Graves' disease will experience some degree of eye problems, although they may be only minor irritations. More serious symptoms can be treated and usually settle in time

■ Agranulocytosis (reduction in white blood cells causing severe sore throat) is a medical emergency and you must contact your doctor immediately and insist on an appointment that day

Underactive thyroid

What is an underactive thyroid?

An underactive thyroid (hypothyroidism) occurs when the thyroid gland stops producing enough of the thyroid hormones, triiodothyronine or T_3 and thyroxine or T_4. In its most common form, affecting one per cent of the population, mainly middle-aged and elderly women, the thyroid gland shrinks as its cells are all destroyed by a subtle defect in the patient's immune system.

Less often this defect leads not only to hypothyroidism but to thyroid enlargement and the formation of a goitre. This is known as Hashimoto's thyroiditis. These types of hypothyroidism are associated, as is Graves' disease, with the other so-called 'autoimmune diseases' (see Glossary, page 102) shown in the box on page 39.

Although having hypothyroidism makes you more likely to develop one or more of these conditions than other people, the risk is still small. The other reason why people develop hypothyroidism is as a result of treatment of Graves' disease by surgery or with radioactive iodine.

What is the pattern of development?

Hypothyroidism does not come on overnight but slowly over many months and you and your family may not notice the symptoms at first, or may simply put them down to ageing.

GPs now have ready access to the appropriate laboratory tests and, as a result, hypothyroidism is increasingly likely to be diagnosed at a relatively early stage when symptoms are mild. Hypothyroidism in its advanced state is sometimes known as 'myxoedema'.

It would be unusual to have all the symptoms mentioned on pages 40–1 unless the diagnosis had been delayed for some reason for months or even

Autoimmune diseases associated with hypothyroidism

- Pernicious anaemia for which regular injections of vitamin B_{12} are necessary to maintain a normal blood count
- Diabetes mellitus usually requiring treatment with insulin
- Addison's disease: the adrenal glands which sit on top of each kidney produce insufficient cortisol and aldosterone, hormones that fortunately can be taken as tablets
- Premature ovarian failure which causes loss of periods, infertility and an early menopause
- Underactivity of the glands adjacent to the thyroid, the parathyroid glands, leads to a low level of calcium in the blood and tetany which is effectively treated with vitamin D capsules
- Vitiligo, a skin disease in which there are areas of loss of pigmentation, gives a 'piebald' appearance

years. You're more likely to go to your GP with rather vague complaints such as tiredness and weight gain, which could be due to a variety of causes.

You'll have a blood test and, if the result shows that you have low T_4 and high thyroid-stimulating hormone (TSH) levels, this will be confirmation that you are suffering from hypothyroidism. Unless there is a complication, such as angina, you will be treated by your family doctor.

Symptoms of hypothyroidism
Weight gain
Most patients gain from five kilograms to ten kilograms, although your appetite is normal or even less than usual.

Sensitivity to the cold
You'll feel the cold very badly, and want to wear extra layers of clothing and sit close to the fire. You may well suffer from muscle stiffness and spasm when you move suddenly, especially when it's cold.

Mental problems
Tiredness, sleepiness and slowing down intellectually. Your reactions get slow, but, fortunately, your sense of humour is unaffected.

Older patients may be wrongly thought to be suffering from dementia, while some people experience depression and paranoia, which are the basis for what is popularly known as 'myxoedema madness'.

Speech
Your voice becomes slow and husky and speech is often slurred.

Heart

In contrast to a person with an overactive thyroid gland, your pulse rate is slow at around 60 beats per minute. You may have high blood pressure and an elderly patient with severe long-standing hypothyroidism is at risk of heart failure. Angina may be the first symptom of hypothyroidism.

Bowel movements

You probably suffer from constipation.

Menstruation

Your periods become heavier (menorrhagia) if you haven't yet had your menopause.

Skin and hair

Your skin is likely to be rough and dry and to flake readily. It tends to be pale and your eyelids, hands and feet swell. Some people may find that their skin has a lemon-yellowish tint and prominent blood vessels in the cheeks add a purplish flush.

Sitting too close to the fire can cause a 'granny's tartan' to appear on the skin of your legs. Some people get the skin condition known as vitiligo. Your hair becomes dry and brittle and the outer part of your eyebrows may be missing.

Nervous system

You may become a little deaf and have trouble with your balance. If your fingers tingle, especially during the night, shaking your hands vigorously should relieve it.

Confirming the diagnosis

This requires a simple blood test to measure the levels

of T_4, which will be low, and TSH, which will be high. If these results are borderline, the measurement of antibodies directed against the thyroid (peroxidase antibodies) will tell whether you have underlying thyroid disease that may justify treatment with T_4 or whether your results, although at the extreme end of the reference range, are normal for you.

Treatment

This is with thyroxine (likely to be written as levothyroxine on a prescription) which is available in the UK as 25, 50 and 100 microgram tablets. Normally, thyroxine treatment is begun slowly and you'll be prescribed a daily dose of 50 micrograms for 3 to 4 weeks, increasing to 100 micrograms daily.

You'll then have another blood test some three months after starting treatment to assess whether any further minor adjustment of dose is necessary. The aim is to restore levels of T_4 and TSH in the blood to normal.

You should start to feel better within two to three weeks; you'll lose weight and notice the puffiness around your eyes disappearing quite soon, but your skin and hair texture may take three to six months to recover fully. Normally you'll have to expect to stay on thyroxine treatment for life.

Very rarely, patients who have had an underactive thyroid for years develop an overactive gland as a result of Graves' disease.

Case history

Jean Spencer was 17 and in her final year at school, hoping to go to university to study law. She had had diabetes since she was 11 and gave herself insulin injections twice each day.

Treatment for an underactive thyroid gland (hypothyroidism)

Before
The thyroid gland produces inadequate amounts of thyroid hormones

After
Thyroxine taken by mouth supplements the low thyroid hormones and is converted by the body to the active hormone T_3

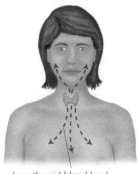

Low thyroid blood level

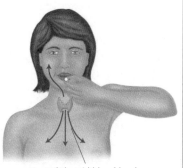

Normal thyroid blood level

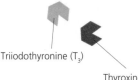

Triiodothyronine (T_3)

Thyroxine (T_4)

Control of her diabetes had always been very satisfactory and her dose of insulin did not vary much. She had been puzzled, however, for the last three months because she did not seem to require as much insulin as before. On four occasions she had almost become unconscious in class because of a low level of glucose in her blood but had been brought round with sugary drinks by her teacher.

Once she did not respond and was rushed to hospital and given a glucose drip into a vein and kept in overnight. Jean's parents and her teacher were also concerned because she was not concentrating in class and her results in the mock exams had not been nearly as good as expected. She had also begun to complain of the cold and had not been able to sing in the school Christmas concert because her voice had become husky.

It was her aunt, visiting from Canada, who recognised the change in Jean's appearance since her visit the previous year. The aunt had developed an underactive thyroid gland 10 years earlier and suggested to Jean that she have a blood test. Jean is now taking thyroxine tablets, like her aunt, and her insulin dose has returned to its previous level. She passed her A levels with flying colours and is now in her first term at university studying law.

Special situations
Angina
The level of various fats or lipids in the blood is increased in hypothyroidism and, in people who have had the condition unrecognised for a long time, the coronary arteries can become narrowed by fatty deposits, a process called atherosclerosis. Insufficient blood reaches the heart muscle, especially during exercise, and the sufferer will get pain in the middle of the chest (angina).

Treatment with thyroxine may worsen the angina and someone with this problem will be started on a lower dose and have it increased more slowly than normal. It may be necessary to have an operation to improve the blood flow through the coronary arteries before or after starting thyroxine treatment.

The process of atherosclerosis

Atherosclerosis, atheroma and hardening of the arteries are all the same thing – the process leading to the blockage or weakening of arteries.

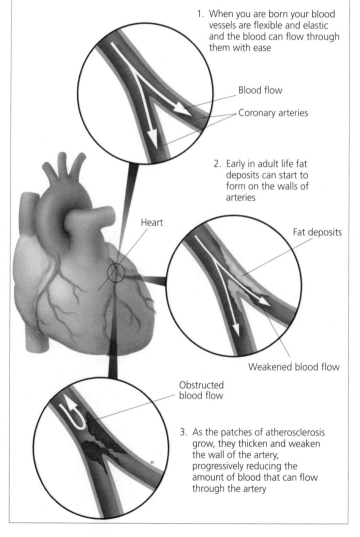

1. When you are born your blood vessels are flexible and elastic and the blood can flow through them with ease

Blood flow

Coronary arteries

2. Early in adult life fat deposits can start to form on the walls of arteries

Fat deposits

Heart

Weakened blood flow

Obstructed blood flow

3. As the patches of atherosclerosis grow, they thicken and weaken the wall of the artery, progressively reducing the amount of blood that can flow through the artery

Temporary hypothyroidism

Treatment with thyroxine is usually for life. However, if you develop hypothyroidism in the first three to four months after surgery or radioactive iodine treatment for Graves' disease it may be short-lived, lasting only a few weeks, and you may not need any treatment. The same is true for the hypothyroidism that is a complication of postpartum (after childbirth) thyroiditis (see page 58) or de Quervain's thyroiditis (see page 32).

Mild hypothyroidism

Most GPs will arrange for someone to have a blood test even when they only suspect thyroid problems, so quite minor abnormalities are often picked up in patients who come because of a variety of rather vague symptoms, such as tiredness, or in people who have a family history of autoimmune disease.

The most common finding is the combination of a 'normal' T_4 but raised TSH level, known among doctors as subclinical hypothyroidism. It is known that around 5 to 20 per cent of these people will develop more obvious hypothyroidism in each following year.

For this reason, it is now common practice to 'nip things in the bud' by prescribing thyroxine when the abnormality has been found on more than one occasion. This may not have any dramatic effect on the individual concerned, but preventive medicine is better than cure.

Hypothyroidism caused by drugs

One drug, called lithium carbonate, which is widely used for depression and mania, may cause goitre and hypothyroidism. When, as normally happens, a person needs to keep taking lithium carbonate, continued treatment with thyroxine will be necessary.

Amiodarone, used in the treatment of certain heart irregularities, may cause not only hyperthyroidism but also hypothyroidism and anyone who is taking it will need regular thyroid blood tests.

Change to your usual dose of thyroxine

The dose of thyroxine may need to be increased during pregnancy (pages 51–60), if there is malabsorption of food by the bowel, such as in coeliac disease, or lack of acid secretion by the stomach as in pernicious anaemia or while taking anti-ulcer drugs, such as omeprazole. There is an increasing list of medicines that reduce the absorption of thyroxine or speed up its breakdown by the body. If you need more thyroxine, the TSH level will increase significantly, having previously been normal.

Thyroxine is now manufactured in the UK by a variety of companies. This is known as generic thyroxine and, despite rigorous controls, doctors and patients have noticed from blood test results and from symptoms that there may be a variation in tablet strength between different manufacturers. For this reason, it is wise to insist that the same make of thyroxine is dispensed by the pharmacist when you renew the prescription. If it is not possible to provide the same make, you should consider having a blood test some six to eight weeks after starting the new preparation.

Possible future treatment

Most patients with hypothyroidism feel perfectly well while taking an appropriate amount of thyroxine, as judged by measurement of T_4 and TSH in the blood. However, some patients do not achieve the sense of well-being expected, even if a little extra thyroxine is taken, which results in a low rather than a normal TSH level.

Commonly prescribed drugs that may increase the need for thyroxine

Drug	Use
Carbamazepine (Tegretol)	Control of epilepsy
Sertraline (Lustral)	Antidepressant
Ferrous sulphate (Feospan, Ferrograd)	Treatment of anaemia
The pill, hormone replacement treatment	Contraception, menopausal symptoms
Chloroquine (Avloclor, Nivaquine)	Antimalarial
Calcium	Osteoporosis
Proton pump inhibitors (Losec, Zoton, Nexium)	Treatment of peptic ulcer and gastro-oesophageal reflux (heartburn)

If you are one of this small group of patients, there is some evidence that a combination of thyroxine and the other thyroid hormone, T_3 (triiodothyronine), may be beneficial.

If you change to this combined treatment, the dose of thyroxine should be reduced by 25–50 micrograms and half a tablet (10 micrograms) of T_3, also known as liothyronine, added. This combination treatment should be supervised by a specialist. If there is still no improvement in well-being, despite normal blood levels of T_3, T_4 and TSH, other causes should be identified for your symptoms and any possibility that the thyroid is in some way responsible dismissed.

Some patients have turned to an old-fashioned medicine, thyroid extract, made from the thyroid gland of animals, which contains both T_3 and T_4 (Armour thyroid). These tablets are not readily available in the UK and, because of continuing anxieties about the reliability of their hormone content, their use is not recommended.

It makes sense to replace what is missing when the thyroid gland stops working and the ideal replacement tablet would contain about 100 micrograms T_4 and 10 micrograms T_3, the latter in a slow-release form. This would avoid peak levels of T_3 in the blood after taking the medication, which can produce troublesome palpitations. Unfortunately such an ideal medicine has not yet been produced by the pharmaceutical industry.

KEY POINTS

■ Hypothyroidism usually comes on slowly and your symptoms are likely to be vague at first

■ Your GP will be able to confirm the diagnosis with a simple blood test

■ Treatment is with tablets, which you'll probably need to take for the rest of your life

■ Some people who have been hypothyroid for many years may suffer from chest pain caused by angina and, because thyroxine aggravates the problem, their dosage will need careful monitoring. If you already have angina when your thyroid condition is first discovered, your treatment will be adjusted to take account of this

■ If your thyroid blood test is only slightly abnormal, you may be given preventive treatment with thyroxine

Thyroid disease and pregnancy

Graves' disease and pregnancy

Hyperthyroidism occurring during pregnancy is almost always the result of Graves' disease. It is not a common event, however, as autoimmune diseases (see Glossary, page 102), of which Graves' disease is an example, tend to improve of their own accord during pregnancy. Also, women with an overactive thyroid gland are relatively infertile because there is an increase in the number of menstrual cycles during which an egg is not released from the ovaries.

As the thyroid-stimulating antibody responsible for the hyperthyroidism of Graves' disease crosses the placenta and passes from the blood of the mother to that of the developing child, it too will have an overactive thyroid gland like its mother. Fortunately, the antithyroid drugs also cross the placenta and good control of hyperthyroidism in the mother will ensure that the fetus comes to no harm. Failure to recognise

The placenta

The fetus is reliant on the mother for oxygen and nutrients.
The placenta allows the exchange of oxygen and nourishment
between the mother and the fetus.

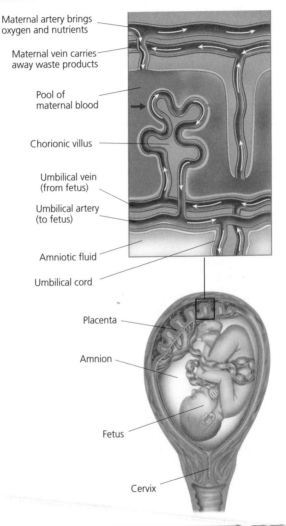

Maternal artery brings oxygen and nutrients

Maternal vein carries away waste products

Pool of maternal blood

Chorionic villus

Umbilical vein (from fetus)

Umbilical artery (to fetus)

Amniotic fluid

Umbilical cord

Placenta

Amnion

Fetus

Cervix

hyperthyroidism or to treat it adequately in a pregnant woman may lead to miscarriage. Overtreatment with antithyroid drugs may lead to goitre development in the fetus. It is important, therefore, that the patient is prescribed the lowest dose of carbimazole possible to restore thyroid hormone levels in the blood to normal. These levels are checked every four to six weeks, in close cooperation with the obstetrician who is caring for her.

The carbimazole is usually stopped four weeks before the expected date of delivery to make sure that there is no possibility of the fetus being hypothyroid at a crucial time in its development.

If hyperthyroidism recurs in the mother after the baby is born, and she is breast-feeding, she will be treated with propylthiouracil rather than carbimazole because it is excreted in the breast milk much less and will not therefore affect the baby.

There are some reports from North America that carbimazole is associated with a rare disease in the newborn baby, known as aplasia cutis, in which there is a defect in the skin covering a small part of the scalp. The view in the UK is, however, that the risk has been overestimated, if it is present at all.

Most specialists in this country are happy to prescribe carbimazole during pregnancy. Some, however, may prefer to use propylthiouracil and to change from carbimazole before conception, if possible. The dose of propylthiouracil is ten times that of carbimazole, and it is available as 50 milligram tablets only.

Radioactive iodine treatment is never given during pregnancy. Surgery is occasionally advised around week 20 of pregnancy for patients who develop side effects to the drugs or who take them irregularly, thereby putting the fetus at risk.

Hyperthyroidism in the newborn (neonatal thyrotoxicosis)

In most women with Graves' disease during pregnancy, the thyroid-stimulating antibody disappears or its level in the blood becomes low. In some, however, the level remains high and, as blood from the mother is exchanged with that of the fetus until the moment of birth, these high levels are also present in the blood of the newborn and may cause hyperthyroidism. Although it is possible to predict those babies most likely to develop hyper-thyroidism by finding high levels of antibodies in the mother's blood towards the end of pregnancy, all newborns in the UK have a blood test shortly after birth to check thyroid hormone levels.

Hyperthyroidism in the newborn, if detected at this stage, is easily treated and lasts only two to three weeks until the antibody from the mother is broken down and inactivated. Very occasionally, mothers who have been treated successfully for Graves' disease in the past continue to produce thyroid-stimulating antibody and their offspring are at risk of developing neonatal hyperthyroidism.

Case history

Rebecca and her husband had been trying to have a second child for three years without success. Rebecca had conceived twice but, unfortunately, on each occasion had miscarried at about ten weeks. She felt and looked well and, although she had lost a few pounds in weight, she put this down to her busy lifestyle of running the home, looking after an active five-year-old son, and working part-time as a secretary. She was a little anxious that her periods, which used to be as regular as clockwork, had become much lighter and, on occasion, were missing.

During her weekly telephone call to her mother, she learned that her cousin in Australia had recently been diagnosed as having an overactive thyroid gland. She consulted her GP and, despite her lack of obvious signs and having neither a goitre nor bulging eyes, the blood test showed the presence of mild hyperthyroidism and this was confirmed as being caused by Graves' disease at the local hospital. Treatment was started with carbimazole, initially in a dose of 30 milligrams daily and, after five months of treatment, Rebecca was pregnant.

She was reviewed by the endocrinologist every four weeks and, by the middle of her pregnancy, she needed to take only five milligrams of carbimazole every day. The drug was stopped four weeks before the expected date of delivery and she gave birth to a healthy girl whose heel-prick blood test at seven days was normal, with no evidence of thyroid abnormality. Rebecca breast-fed her daughter but, after four months, developed hyperthyroidism, again as a result of Graves' disease because the thyroid-stimulating antibody was present in her blood. She decided to change to bottle-feeding and her hyperthyroidism was therefore treated with carbimazole as before. Had she opted to continue breast-feeding, propylthiouracil would have been prescribed instead.

Hypothyroidism and pregnancy

Most women with hypothyroidism are already taking thyroxine when they become pregnant. Although mild hypothyroidism is unlikely to affect fertility, women with severe thyroid deficiency of prolonged duration are unlikely to become pregnant and, if they conceive, to maintain their pregnancy.

The dose of thyroxine may need to be increased in pregnancy. Recent research shows that the increase is most important to the fetus in early pregnancy. As soon as you become pregnant visit your doctor who will probably increase your thyroxine dose by 25 micrograms and carry out a blood test. You will be tested every two months or so during pregnancy and the average extra dose of thyroxine needed will be 50 micrograms daily. You can return to the dose you were taking before pregnancy after your baby has been born.

Although the thyroid gland of the fetus develops independently of the mother and makes its own thyroid hormones, a recent study in the USA has shown that unrecognised or inadequately treated hypothyroidism in the mother may cause a slight reduction in the IQ of the child. Your baby will not be at risk if you forget the occasional dose, but if you make a habit of not taking it, not only will you face a greater risk of miscarriage, but your baby may not be as intelligent as he or she might have been.

It would be sensible for those taking thyroxine or those who have a family history of thyroid disease to check that their thyroid blood tests are normal when planning a pregnancy, and therefore before conception.

Hypothyroidism in the newborn (congenital hypothyroidism)

One in about 3,500 newborn babies has an underactive thyroid gland as a result of failure of the gland to develop normally. In the past, the problem was not recognised until the child was several weeks old, by which time he or she would have been likely to develop permanent mental and physical handicap – the condition known then as cretinism. Today, however, all

Heel-prick test
Heel-prick blood test on new baby.

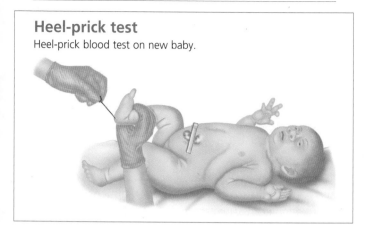

newborn babies are screened by a blood test for hypothyroidism between five and seven days after they are born. Any affected children are given prompt treatment which ensures that they develop normally.

Treatment is usually for life, but in a few babies the hypothyroidism is temporary as a result of being born to a mother with an underactive thyroid gland; in these women there are blocking antibodies that cross the placenta and have the opposite effect of the stimulating antibodies of Graves' disease and neonatal thyrotoxicosis (see page 54).

Thyroid disease after pregnancy
Although the hyperthyroidism of Graves' disease tends to get better on its own during pregnancy, it often returns in a severe form within a few months of delivery. There is, however, another form of hyperthyroidism that may develop in the first year after childbirth, almost always in patients who have an underlying autoimmune thyroid disease such as Hashimoto's thyroiditis, which may not have been recognised previously.

The hyperthyroidism is mild and lasts only a few weeks; if treatment is neccessary, only a beta blocker is taken. This phase may be followed by an equally transient episode of mild hypothyroidism not requiring treatment, and then usually by full recovery. A similar pattern may occur in future pregnancies and many patients ultimately develop a permanently underactive thyroid.

To distinguish between what is known as postpartum thyroiditis (see Glossary, page 102), not requiring treatment, and Graves' disease, which requires treatment, two measurements may be necessary. One is the concentration of thyroid-stimulating antibody in the blood, as this is usually present in Graves' disease. The other is the ability of the thyroid gland to concentrate radioactive iodine or technetium, as this is lacking in postpartum thyroiditis.

Postpartum thyroiditis affects about five per cent of women but most patients do not complain of symptoms. There does not appear to be any association between the thyroid blood test abnormalities and postnatal depression.

Case history

Flora Stewart was 25 and happily married to her lawyer husband, William, and they had had their first child, Jane, five months earlier. Their relationship began to deteriorate when Flora became weepy and short-tempered, snapping at William for no good reason. She was also sleeping badly and William noticed that Flora's hands sometimes trembled.

However, they both put all this down to hormonal changes following her pregnancy and the birth of their baby, and assumed that before long everything would be back to normal. When Flora began to complain of palpitations, William persuaded her to visit their GP.

The doctor thought that Flora might have an overactive thyroid gland and his suspicions were confirmed by a blood test.

On hearing the news Flora was concerned because her mother had suffered from Graves' disease when she was in her 30s and her eyes were still very prominent 20 years later, even though the hyperthyroidism had been cured. In order to relieve some of Flora's symptoms her GP prescribed a long-acting form of propranolol (Inderal LA) 80 milligrams, to be taken once daily and he suggested that Flora should see a specialist at the local hospital. By the time her appointment came round four weeks later, Flora felt much better and a repeat blood sample showed that her thyroid gland had become very slightly underactive.

The diagnosis was not that of Graves' disease, but of postpartum thyroiditis, and Flora was reassured that she would not get bulging eyes like her mother. The propranolol was stopped, and another blood test two months later was entirely normal.

Flora now knows that she may get the symptoms of postpartum thyroiditis after further pregnancies, and that she has an increased chance of developing a permanently underactive thyroid gland at some stage in the future.

However, her GP will do a thyroid blood test every year to make sure that it is detected before she can develop severe symptoms.

KEY POINTS

■ There is no reason why you cannot become pregnant while taking an antithyroid drug for Graves' disease, but you do need to be closely supervised by a specialist, together with your obstetrician, throughout your pregnancy

■ If you are taking thyroxine and become pregnant, the dose should be increased immediately by 25 micrograms and a blood test arranged with your GP in three to four weeks.

■ Some women will develop mild thyroid disease after having a baby, but this is easily treated. If you are experiencing similar symptoms to those described in Flora's story on page 58, it is worth asking your GP whether this could be the cause

■ Although your child may be born with hypothyroidism or hyperthyroidism, if you suffer from either condition, like all newborns he or she will be given a routine test shortly after birth and treated if necessary

Enlarged thyroid

Development of a goitre

An enlarged thyroid gland is known as a goitre. There are many causes, including a shortage of iodine in the diet which occurs in remote mountainous parts of the world, drugs such as lithium carbonate (Priadel) used to treat patients with bipolar disorder, and autoimmune disorders such as Hashimoto's thyroiditis (see page 38) and Graves' disease (see page 8).

The cause of most goitres in this country is not known, however. Such goitres are called 'simple goitres' despite the fact that there are almost certainly complex reasons for their development. Although the thyroid gland is enlarged it continues to produce normal amounts of hormones and the patient is referred to as 'euthyroid' as opposed to hyperthyroid or hypothyroid.

At first, in teenagers and young adults, the goitre is evenly or diffusely enlarged. During the next 15 to 25 years, whatever caused the thyroid to grow abnormally in the first place remains and it continues to grow but becomes full of lumps or nodules. By the time the young person reaches middle age, the goitre will have become lumpy, when it is known medically as a 'multinodular goitre'.

Simple diffuse goitre

Most of those who have a simple diffuse goitre are young women between the ages of 15 and 25. If you are one of them, you (or your relatives) will have noticed a symmetrical, smooth swelling in the front of your neck. You may have had it for some years but thought it was just 'puppy fat'. The goitre will move up and down when you swallow. It is not tender, however, and does not usually cause difficulty in swallowing but you may experience a tight sensation in your neck.

The goitre may vary slightly in size and be more noticeable at the time of a period or during pregnancy. It isn't normally a problem appearance-wise – quite the opposite as far as some people are concerned. For example, the great seventeenth and eighteenth century artists often added a goitre to the female figure to enhance her beauty!

Confirming the diagnosis

Usually your GP will want you to be seen by a specialist to exclude the rarer causes of goitre. He or she can normally do this by feeling your neck and by taking blood tests.

Treatment

No treatment is necessary. In the past iodine (often added to milk) or thyroxine tablets were given but neither is effective. Many people find that their goitre becomes less noticeable or even disappears over a period of two to three years.

Simple multinodular goitre

If you are in your 40s or 50s, you will probably first become aware of a swelling in your neck while washing or applying make-up in front of a mirror. In fact, the goitre will have been present for many years but has now reached a critical size, or it may be that your neck has become thinner.

The goitre is often more obvious on one side of the neck than the other. It may vary in size from being barely visible to other people to so large that you feel you have to hide it by wearing scarves or high-necked sweaters.

A few people notice the enlarged thyroid gland for the first time because internal bleeding causes increased swelling which is accompanied by discomfort in the neck, like a bruise, lasting a few days.

If the goitre is large there may be difficulty in swallowing dry, solid food and, if the trachea (windpipe) is squashed to any extent, there may be difficulty in breathing; singers, in particular, will notice a change in their voice.

Confirming the diagnosis

Your GP may take a blood sample to check that your thyroid hormone levels are normal but will usually ask a specialist for advice about further investigations and treatment. The specialist may wish to carry out one or more of the following tests.

X-ray and breathing tests

These will reveal whether the goitre is compressing or squashing the windpipe.

Ultrasound scan

A probe, the size of a small hand torch, is passed over

Investigations

You may have further investigations to confirm your diagnosis.

X-ray investigation

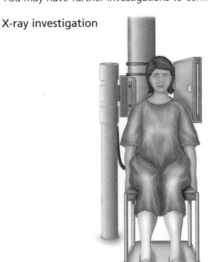

Ultrasound scan

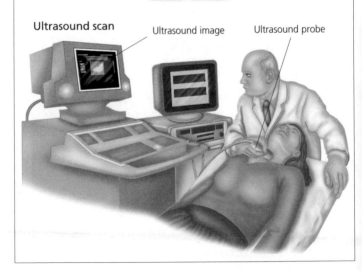

Ultrasound image

Ultrasound probe

the skin of the front of the neck and an image of the goitre is formed on a screen. As well as showing its size and extent it will also highlight any cysts or nodules that the specialist may not have noticed by examining the neck.

Isotope scan

This technique provides a different type of image which shows whether the nodules in the goitre are likely to be producing thyroid hormones, in which case the development of an overactive thyroid is more likely in future years. It is obtained by injecting a tiny amount of radioactivity in the form of a radioactive substance called technetium-99m into a vein. About half an hour after the injection you lie under a sophisticated form of camera for a few minutes (see page 17).

Fine needle aspiration

This involves attaching a needle of the same size as that used for taking a blood sample to the end of a syringe, then, while you're lying down, passing it without local anaesthetic through the skin of the neck into the enlarged thyroid gland. If the nodule is very small, the procedure may be carried out with the help of ultrasound to ensure that the needle is in the correct place.

The discomfort is no more than that felt during straightforward blood tests. By pulling on the plunger and moving the needle up and down a tiny distance within the goitre, the doctor can obtain thyroid cells for analysis.

These are smeared on to a glass slide and, after processing in the pathology laboratory, are examined under a microscope. The appearance of the cells will help to determine whether the thyroid enlargement is the result of a malignant tumour.

Fine needle aspiration

The doctor extracts cells from the thyroid gland using a syringe with a fine needle.

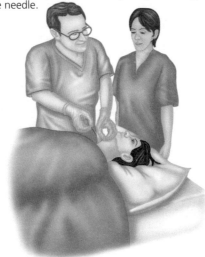

Fine needle

Vacuum in syringe

Lump in gland

Trachea (windpipe)

Inside the neck

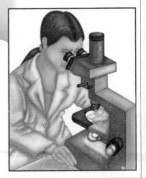

The sample is processed in a laboratory and examined under a microscope for abnormalities

Fine needle aspiration, commonly known as FNA, is not often carried out in patients with a multinodular goitre unless the gland is very much bigger on one side than the other, or the goitre is growing very rapidly.

Treatment

If your goitre is relatively small, you probably won't need any treatment. Your GP will check thyroid hormone levels in your blood every one to two years as there is a possibility of the gland becoming overactive and causing hyperthyroidism at some stage during the next 20 years or so. Although thyroxine tablets are prescribed in certain parts of the world in an attempt to shrink the goitre, they are of little or no benefit and may cause hyperthyroidism.

Surgery

If the goitre becomes so large that it looks really unattractive or is compressing the windpipe, the most effective treatment is an operation to remove most of the thyroid gland. No treatment is necessary before surgery and you'll be in hospital for about three days. The complications are the same as those for surgery for Graves' disease (page 20). You may have to take thyroxine treatment afterwards as there may be insufficient thyroid tissue left to produce adequate amounts of hormones.

Radioactive iodine

In patients who aren't fit enough for surgery or who don't want to have an operation, it may be possible to reduce the size of the goitre by about 50 per cent by giving radioactive iodine. A large dose is necessary, and you may have to be admitted to hospital for 24 to 48 hours.

The possible change of a goitre over a lifetime

The smooth so-called simple goitre of young adulthood changes to the multinodular goitre of middle age and the toxic multinodular goitre of old age. The cause of the goitre is not known but, if whatever makes the thyroid gland grow in the first place continues to be present, the thyroid develops lumps or nodules. These nodules make their own thyroid hormones and, as they increase in number and size over many years, hyperthyroidism develops. The windpipe (trachea), shown by the dotted lines, may be displaced and narrowed as the goitre enlarges.

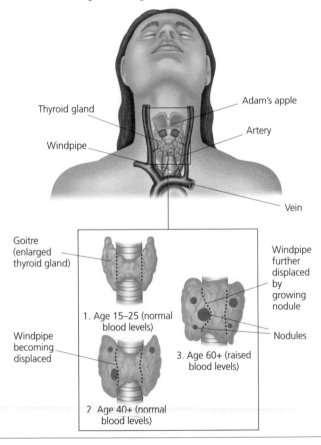

Thyroid gland

Adam's apple

Artery

Windpipe

Vein

Goitre (enlarged thyroid gland)

Windpipe further displaced by growing nodule

Windpipe becoming displaced

Nodules

1. Age 15–25 (normal blood levels)

3. Age 60+ (raised blood levels)

2. Age 40+ (normal blood levels)

If so, you'll be given a single room to avoid contaminating other patients and visitors with radioactivity.

It may take several months for the goitre to shrink. It is unlikely that the thyroid will become underactive because the radioactive iodine is mainly concentrated within the nodules and, as they become smaller, the thyroid tissue surrounding them that has been dormant and unaffected by the radiation wakes up and starts to produce thyroid hormones.

Case history

Jenny Morris was a single woman in her seventies who had been an accomplished actress. She always wore a silk scarf around her neck, day and night, summer and winter. Friends and neighbours thought it was part of her slightly eccentric personality, but when she was admitted to hospital as an emergency with abdominal pain due to gallstones the scarf was removed to reveal a large goitre and a scar from a previous thyroid operation.

Miss Morris explained that the operation had been carried out for a goitre when she was quite young. In her mid-forties the goitre appeared again but she was told further surgery was out of the question because a second operation was technically more difficult and any damage to the nearby nerve supply to the voice box (larynx) would ruin her stage career. As time passed the goitre gradually grew and grew, and she took to wearing the scarves to avoid embarrassment.

Blood tests in hospital showed her to have a slightly overactive thyroid gland and three months after treatment with radioactive iodine her blood test came back normal. Equally important, a year later, the size of the goitre had been reduced by at least a half, and she happily abandoned her scarves!

Thyroid nodules

Single lumps or nodules in the thyroid are common,
and can occur at any age. Women are more likely to be
affected than men.

A single thyroid nodule

The nodule varies in size from that of a pea to a golf
ball or even larger. Like a goitre, the nodule is usually
discovered by accident while you're washing or looking
in a mirror. Bleeding into the nodule may cause pain
which alerts you to its presence. The discomfort usually
lasts two to three days and often, by the time that you
have seen a specialist, the nodule will have shrunk or
even disappeared.

Alternatively, the nodule may be discovered during
medical examination for some quite unrelated problem,
although neither you nor your family had noticed it
before. Most women are aware of the significance of
a lump in the breast, and so naturally suspect that a
nodule in the thyroid may also mean cancer. This is why
your GP will probably want you to see a specialist. In
fact, the great majority of single thyroid nodules are
not cancers of the thyroid.

Confirming the diagnosis

If you have a single thyroid nodule, your blood test will
show normal levels of T_3, T_4 and TSH, which means
you're classified medically as 'euthyroid'; the exception
is the 'toxic adenoma' in which the thyroid blood tests
will demonstrate an overactive thyroid gland.

The thyroid specialist will wish to examine your
neck carefully as about half of all patients thought
to have a single nodule are in fact found to have
generalised nodular enlargement of the thyroid known

as multinodular goitre. In this case you can be assured that your condition is not serious.

Those people who need further investigations may have an X-ray, ultrasound or radioisotope scan of their thyroid, but the single most important test is fine needle aspiration (FNA) of the lump.

The technique is simple, quick and, if necessary, can be carried out two or three times as it doesn't cause pain or undue discomfort. FNA is one of the most important advances in the care of people with thyroid disease. In the past the majority of those with a single thyroid nodule had to have surgery but many operations can now be avoided simply by examining a small sample of thyroid cells obtained by aspiration in the outpatient clinic. The outcome will be one of those indicated opposite.

Benign (non-cancerous) nodules may continue to enlarge over many years and eventually may get so big that an operation is needed to remove them for the sake of your appearance.

If you can't help worrying about the possibility that the lump is harbouring a cancer, your specialist may well suggest operating to remove the nodule so that it can be examined microscopically and resolve the question once and for all.

What are the possible outcomes of fine needle aspiration (FNA)?

- The needle will remove fluid and the nodule will disappear: this means that the nodule must have been a thyroid cyst and no further treatment is needed. Should the cyst recur it can be aspirated once more but, if it comes back yet again, you will need an operation to remove that half of the thyroid containing the cyst.

- The cells removed from the nodule show that it is a benign lump and therefore you don't have cancer. Unless the swelling is sufficiently large to be disfiguring, when surgery would be necessary, you can be reassured that no treatment is needed.

- The cells removed are malignant which means that the nodule is thyroid cancer, and you will need an immediate operation.

- Sometimes, because of the small number of cells removed, it may be impossible to be certain whether the nodule is benign or malignant (cancer). In this case, you will need an operation to remove the entire nodule so that it can be examined carefully under the microscope.

KEY POINTS

■ In this country, the cause of a goitre usually remains a mystery

■ Young people with a simple diffuse goitre rarely need any treatment

■ You'll probably be referred to a specialist to have a multinodular goitre investigated, and you may have several tests

■ A small goitre may be left alone, but you'll have regular blood tests done by your GP as there's a chance of developing hyperthyroidism later on

■ An operation or treatment with radioactive iodine may be necessary if the goitre is causing problems

■ Thyroxine tablets won't help to shrink a goitre, although they are still prescribed in some other countries

■ Although people who develop thyroid nodules often worry that the lump may be cancer, this rarely turns out to be the case

■ The simple and painless investigation known as fine needle aspiration means that far fewer people now have to have surgery

■ If you're concerned about your appearance or can't stop worrying about the possibility of cancer, you can have an operation to remove the nodule

Thyroid cancer

What is cancer?

A lump of human tissue the size of a sugar cube may contain a thousand million cells. These are the minute building blocks from which our bodies are made, visible only down the microscope. It is quite amazing that the billions of cells in a human body normally function in perfect harmony, every cell knowing its place and doing the job that it was designed to do. Most cells have a finite lifespan: millions of new ones are produced every day to replace those lost through old age or wear and tear.

New cells are produced when existing cells divide into two. Except in children, who are growing, there is normally a perfect balance between the numbers of the cells that are dying and those that are dividing. Normally exactly the right amounts of new cells are produced to replace those that are being lost. The control mechanisms involved are exceedingly complex. Loss of control can lead to an excess of cells, resulting in a tumour.

How a tumour forms

A cancerous tumour begins as a single cell. If it is not destroyed by the body's immune system, it will double into two cells, which in turn divide into four and so on.

| Cancerous cell | First doubling | Second doubling |

However, it is important to realise that only a very small minority of tumours are cancerous. Most tumours are localised accumulations of normal or fairly normal cells and are benign. A wart is a common example.

The development of a cancer (malignant tumour) involves a change in the quality of the cells as well as an increase in quantity: they change in both appearance and behaviour. They become more aggressive, destructive and independent of normal cells. They acquire the ability to infiltrate and invade the surrounding tissues.

In some instances the cells may also invade lymphatic and blood vessels and thus spread away from the 'primary' growth to other places. In time these cells may cause the development of secondary growths, known as 'metastases', in the lymph glands and other organs such as lungs, liver and bones.

Malignant tumours of the thyroid gland are rare. For example, a specialist may see 50 to 100 patients with hyperthyroidism caused by Graves' disease for every one with thyroid cancer. The types of cancer that doctors see most frequently are:

- Papillary cancer which usually affects children and young women.

How cancer spreads

Cancerous tumours can spread to distant sites in the body by a process called metastasis. In metastasis the cancerous cell separates from a malignant tumour and travels to a new location in the blood or lymph.

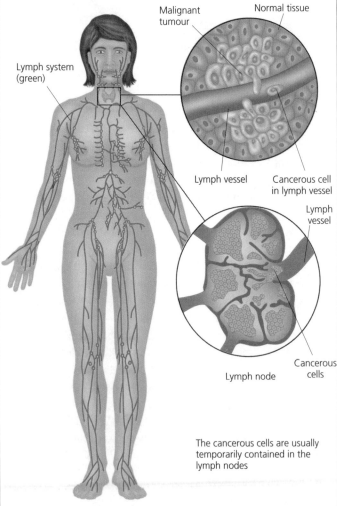

Malignant tumour

Normal tissue

Lymph system (green)

Lymph vessel

Cancerous cell in lymph vessel

Lymph vessel

Lymph node

Cancerous cells

The cancerous cells are usually temporarily contained in the lymph nodes

- Follicular cancer which is unusual before the age of 30.

These terms describe the appearance of the tumour under the microscope. In papillary cancer, the tumour contains papillae or fronds, whereas in follicular cancer, although the appearance is distinctly abnormal, there are still structures that resemble the normal follicles of the thyroid. Both cancers can occur at any age, however.

Provided that diagnosis and treatment are at an early stage, the person may well live out a normal lifespan; in other words, you're still more likely to die of a stroke or a heart attack in old age.

Confirming the diagnosis

Most patients visit their GP with a lump in the neck or because of rapid growth of a goitre that they've had for many years. The diagnosis of thyroid cancer is made at a hospital visit by fine needle aspiration or following surgery.

Occasionally, the patient consults his or her doctor because of enlarged lymph nodes in the neck which may at first be thought to be caused by Hodgkin's disease. However, a biopsy shows that the patient actually has papillary cancer which has spread from the thyroid gland via the lymphatic system to the nearby lymph nodes.

Treatment

Surgery

Both papillary and follicular cancers are usually treated by removing as much of the thyroid gland as possible (total thyroidectomy). Any enlarged lymph nodes in the neck containing thyroid cancer are also removed at this stage.

Microscopic view of the thyroid gland

The follicles seen here in cross-section are best considered as slightly out-of-shape golf balls. The dimples in the surface correspond to the follicle cells that make thyroid hormones and release them into the capillaries, which lie close by. The colloid, where reserves of thyroid hormone are stored, is like the semi-liquid filling of old-fashioned golf balls. There are many thousands of follicles in a thyroid gland. The superimposed needle tip shows that, during fine needle aspiration, a very small sample of cells from two or three follicles is obtained, which may not necessarily give the whole picture.

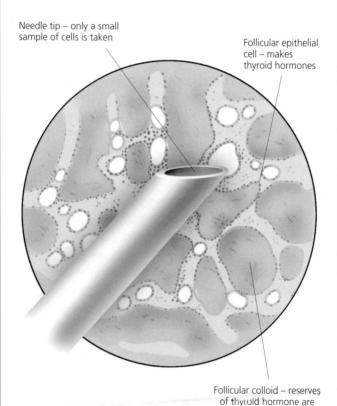

Needle tip – only a small sample of cells is taken

Follicular epithelial cell – makes thyroid hormones

Follicular colloid – reserves of thyroid hormone are stored here

No special treatment is required before the operation and you can usually go home after two days. As a result of the extent of the surgery, damage to the parathyroid glands is more common than in other thyroid surgery.

The low level of calcium in the blood that results is easily treated by taking a vitamin D derivative, known as alfacalcidol (One-Alpha), in a dose of one to two micrograms each day by mouth.

Radioactive iodine

It is not possible to remove every last part of the thyroid gland by means of surgery. For this reason, most patients with papillary or follicular cancer will be given a large dose of radioactive iodine (iodine-131) to kill any remaining cells.

The radioactive iodine is given as a liquid or a capsule in hospital. You will have to stay in hospital for 48 to 72 hours, in a single room, separated from the other patients.

The radioactive iodine is usually given three to four weeks after your operation and before thyroxine tablets have been started, as it is most effective when the patient is hypothyroid and TSH levels in the blood are high. If for some reason there is a delay, and you have already started taking thyroxine to prevent you from becoming hypothyroid after removal of your thyroid gland, you will be taken off the treatment some four weeks before being given the radioactive iodine.

Towards the end of the period without thyroxine you may feel tired but will come to no harm. The thyroxine can be re-started in full dosage 48 hours after your treatment and you will feel your normal self after another 10 to 14 days. An alternative to stopping thyroxine is for Thyrogen (see page 81) to be given by intramuscular injection on each of the two days before the iodine-131 treatment.

Thyroxine

Doctors believe that the rate of growth of papillary and follicular cancers of the thyroid may be increased by the hormone TSH. An important part of the treatment, therefore, is to make sure that you take enough thyroxine to ensure that the level of TSH in your blood becomes undetectable.

Patients with thyroid cancer need a slightly greater dose of thyroxine than those with hypothyroidism. A dose of 150 to 200 micrograms daily is usually sufficient to switch off TSH secretion by the pituitary gland.

Follow-up

Papillary and follicular cancers, like the normal thyroid gland, make a substance called thyroglobulin.

The thyroid gland can secrete this substance only in the presence of TSH, but this is not the case with thyroid cancer. So, if there is no TSH detectable in the bloodstream because it has been suppressed by treatment with thyroxine, any thyroglobulin in the blood must be coming from recurrent cancer in the neck or from cancer that has spread to other parts of the body (secondaries or metastases).

Thyroglobulin is known as a 'tumour marker'. If a patient who is taking appropriate amounts of thyroxine has a raised level of thyroglobulin, the specialist may wish to arrange other tests such as an ultrasound of the neck (see pages 63–5), or a CT scan of the chest to identify the site of the recurrent tumour or its metastases.

Scanning of the whole body using radioactive iodine may also be helpful. The scan is usually performed 24

Computed tomography

Computed tomography (CT) fires X-rays through the body at different angles. The X-rays are picked up by receivers and the information analysed by a computer to create an anatomical picture.

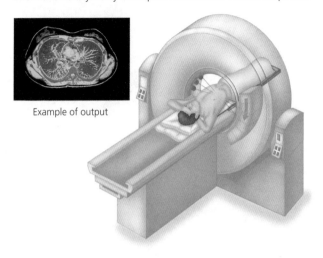

Example of output

to 48 hours after a dose of iodine-131 by mouth, 4 weeks after the patient has stopped taking thyroxine or after TSH (Thyrogen) injections.

Any tumour that is found may be treated with a large dose of radioactive iodine in hospital. PET (positron emission tomography) may be indicated if these imaging tests are negative, but your specialist is suspicious of the continued presence of cancer because of raised levels of the tumour marker, thyroglobulin. A PET scan depends on the more active cancer cells taking up more radioactive glucose than surrounding normal cells after you have been injected with the sugar.

Thyrogen

This is the name given to recombinant human TSH,

Whole body scan

Whole body scan using radioactive iodine and a gamma camera.

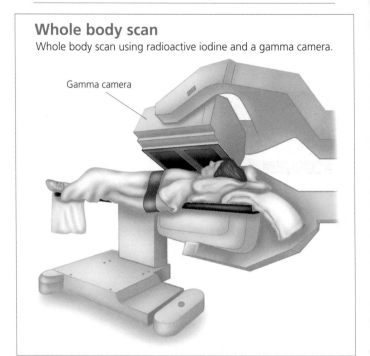

Gamma camera

a protein identical to TSH in the pituitary gland and blood, but which has been made in the laboratory. Thyrogen (thyrotropin alfa) can be given as an intramuscular injection on each of two successive days before whole body scanning or treatment with radioactive iodine.

By increasing the TSH concentrations in the blood in this way, you will not need to stop your thyroxine tablets for four weeks and will not suffer any of the symptoms of an underactive thyroid gland.

Outlook

This depends upon the size of the tumour and whether it has spread at the time of diagnosis. If treated correctly, a young woman with a small papillary cancer of the thyroid is likely to have a normal life expectancy, despite the cancer having spread to the lymph nodes in the neck. Even patients with follicular cancer that has spread to the bones or lungs may survive for many years with a good quality of life.

Case history

Susan Jones was 18 when she fell heavily while skating, striking the side of her neck against the ice-rink barrier. As the pain and bruising settled she noticed a pea-sized lump in her neck. To begin with her doctor thought that it must be related to the accident, although it moved when she swallowed, suggesting that it lay within the thyroid gland rather than in the skin or muscle.

When it hadn't disappeared after six weeks, he referred Susan to a thyroid specialist at the local teaching hospital. The consultant examined Susan's neck carefully and found that, in addition to the single small thyroid nodule, there were three enlarged lymph nodes on the right side of her neck. He proceeded to take a tiny sample from the thyroid nodule and from one of the lymph nodes, sucking out cells with a syringe and needle. The test took only a few minutes, causing Susan no discomfort and with no need even for a local anaesthetic.

The next day Susan and her mother were told that the sample showed that the lump in Susan's neck was a type of cancer of the thyroid, known as papillary carcinoma, and that it had spread to the nearby lymph nodes. The only treatment was an operation and two weeks later Susan was admitted to hospital where almost all of her thyroid gland was removed, together with the enlarged lymph nodes.

Careful inspection of the removed gland by the pathologists showed no other signs of thyroid cancer apart from the original swelling. After the operation, Susan was treated with radioactive iodine to ensure that any remaining thyroid cells had been destroyed.

Susan has been cured and simply needs to take thyroxine tablets for the rest of her life and see the specialist every year for a blood test. The skating accident was a blessing in disguise as it brought to light a thyroid cancer which was at a very early stage. The fact that it had spread to the lymph nodes in the neck was of no consequence.

Rarer cancers

These include the following:

- Medullary cancer of the thyroid which can occur on its own or may run in families in association with abnormalities of other endocrine glands or of the skeleton.

- Lymphoma of the thyroid which usually affects elderly people and may be accompanied by evidence of disease in other parts of the body.

- Anaplastic cancer which also affects elderly people.

The future prospects for people with these types of cancer is less good than for those with papillary or follicular cancer. Treatment is more difficult and may include chemotherapy and radiotherapy.

KEY POINTS

■ Remember that thyroid cancer is rare

■ The two types that doctors see most often – papillary and follicular cancers – can normally be treated successfully if they are caught early enough

■ An operation is necessary to remove as much of the thyroid gland as possible and any abnormal lymph nodes in the neck, followed by treatment with radioactive iodine to destroy any remaining cells

■ After surgery, patients will need to take thyroxine in slightly higher doses than normal

■ A blood test will probably be done after treatment to make sure that there is no trace of cancer remaining and to check that it hasn't spread

■ There are a few very rare cancers which mainly affect elderly people in whom treatment may be more difficult

Thyroid blood tests

Measuring thyroid hormone levels

Increasingly, patients wish to know about the actual levels of thyroid hormones and TSH in the blood. The normal or reference ranges for the commonly measured hormones are shown in the box on page 88.

These ranges will vary slightly from laboratory to laboratory, depending upon the normal population used for the calculations, and upon the type of chemical analysis used for the measurement of the hormones.

The thyroid hormones, triiodothyronine or T_3 and thyroxine or T_4, are almost exclusively bound to a protein in the bloodstream and, as such, are inactive. Less than one per cent of these hormones are unbound or free and able to control the metabolism of the body.

Measurement of total T_3 (TT_3) and T_4 (TT_4) includes both bound and free fractions, whereas measurement of free T_4 (fT_4) and T_3 (fT_3) excludes the much larger bound fraction.

In most circumstances, measurement of free and total thyroid hormones provides the same information about whether the thyroid is working normally or in an over- or underactive fashion. Some hospital laboratories offer the measurement of total thyroid hormones and others of free thyroid hormones, but rarely both.

Typical results in hyperthyroidism and hypothyroidism
Hyperthyroid

Generally speaking, the more severe the symptoms of over- or underactivity of the thyroid gland, the more abnormal the results of the thyroid blood tests. In most patients with hyperthyroidism:

- TT_4 would be about 190 nmol/l
- TT_3 4 nmol/l
- fT_4 40 pmol/l
- fT_3 12 pmol/l.

Much higher values may be recorded, however, with fT_4 in excess of 100 pmol/l. In older patients in whom hyperthyroidism may be no less serious with heart complications, such as an irregular heartbeat caused by atrial fibrillation, the levels of thyroid hormones may be only marginally elevated. In all patients with hyper-thyroidism, with very rare exceptions, the TSH level in the blood is so low that it cannot be detected.

Hypothyroid

By the time that patients with hypothyroidism present with typical symptoms, fT_4 and TT_4 levels are very low and often less than 5 pmol/l and 20 nmol/l respectively, and associated with a raised TSH level in the blood of more than 30 mU/l.

Rarely, hypothyroidism is the result of disease of the pituitary gland and not of the thyroid gland itself,

Normal reference ranges

This table shows the normal reference range of thyroid hormones and TSH in the blood. Your doctor will compare your results with these to assess your condition.

Total thyroxine (TT_4)	60–150 nanomoles per litre (nmol/l)
Free thyroxine (fT_4)	10–25 picomoles per litre (pmol/l)
Total triiodothyronine (TT_3)	1.1–2.6 nanomoles per litre (nmol/l)
Free triiodothyronine (fT_3)	3.0–8.0 picomoles per litre (pmol/l)
Thyrotrophin or thyroid-stimulating hormone (TSH)	0.15–3.5 milliunits per litre (mU/l)

nanomoles = 10^{-9} moles; picomoles = 10^{-12} moles.

For the scientifically minded, a mole is the molecular weight of a substance in grams:

- A mole of thyroxine is 777 grams.

- A nanomole of thyroxine is 777 nanograms (or 777 x 10^{-9} grams)

- A picomole of thyroxine is 777 picograms (or 777 x 10^{-12} grams).

Although most hormones are now measured in molar units, as this is thought to reflect activity more accurately, drugs are still prescribed in mass units or grams. A dose of 100 micrograms (or 100 x 10^{-6} grams) is the equivalent of about 130 nanomoles.

in which case the low fT_4 or TT_4 is combined with a normal or low level of TSH.

In mild or subclinical hypothyroidism (see page 45), fT_4 and TT_4 lie in the lower part of the normal range, for example 11 pmol/l or 65 nmol/l, and are usually associated with a TSH level in the blood of between 5 and 10 mU/l.

Levels of T_3 are not usually measured in patients with suspected hypothyroidism.

Judging the correct dose of thyroxine

Your GP or thyroid specialist will usually prescribe a dose of thyroxine that raises the fT_4 and TT_4 to the upper part of the normal range and reduces the TSH level in the blood to the lower part of the normal range.

Typical results would be a fT_4 of 20 pmol/l or TT_4 of 130 nmol/l, and a TSH of 0.4 mU/l. In some patients, a sense of well-being is not restored, however, and the doctor is often pressurised to sanction an increased dose of thyroxine. Evidence is growing that increasing the dose of thyroxine such that TSH becomes undetectable at less than 0.01 mU/l in the long term may put you at increased risk of future heart disease or osteoporosis. Rather than increase the dose of thyroxine to potentially dangerous levels, it may be sensible to change to a combination of thyroxine and triiodothyronine (liothyronine), ensuring that TSH levels are normal. Such combination treatment requires the supervision initially of a specialist.

Failure to take thyroxine regularly is very obvious from blood test results.

Effect of illness on thyroid blood tests

Illness, whether sudden such as pneumonia or a heart attack, or of long duration, such as rheumatoid arthritis or depression, may affect the results of thyroid blood tests and give the impression of hyper- or hypothyroidism. It is possible that, after referral to a specialist and after further investigations, no underlying thyroid disease will be found.

THYROID BLOOD TESTS SHOULD NOT BE INTERPRETED IN ISOLATION AND CORRECT MEDICAL CARE WILL ALSO DEPEND ON CAREFUL ASSESSMENT OF SYMPTOMS AND CLINICAL EXAMINATION.

KEY POINTS

■ The normal ranges for thyroid blood tests will vary from laboratory to laboratory

■ Generally, the more severe the symptoms the more abnormal the results of the thyroid blood test

■ Thyroid blood tests should not be interpreted in isolation

'Hypothyroidism' with normal blood tests

Some patients are convinced that their symptoms of tiredness, weight gain and feeling low are the result of an underactive thyroid gland, even though levels of the hormones thyroxine (T_4) and thyroid-stimulating hormone (TSH) are normal.

This mistaken belief has not been helped by numerous articles in newspapers and magazines and inaccurate information on the internet. Unfortunately, a few doctors are prepared to diagnose hypothyroidism and treat patients with thyroid hormones, even though blood tests are normal or with no blood testing at all. These doctors do not usually have any training in thyroid disease.

The following answers to questions frequently asked by patients who feel that they would benefit from thyroid hormone treatment may help to convince you that it is not possible to have an underactive thyroid gland if the blood levels of T_4 and TSH are normal.

'But I have the symptoms of an underactive thyroid . . .'

The trouble is that the symptoms of an underactive thyroid gland are what we call non-specific. In other words, similar complaints are also made by patients with other problems. For example, many middle-aged women gain weight and this may lead to tiredness, as may the menopause itself, or there may be stress at home and at work. Most of us feel down from time to time and prolonged fatigue might easily result from a recent viral infection. If thyroid blood tests are normal, it makes no sense to insist that the thyroid can still be underactive, rather than consider other diagnoses, changes in lifestyle, or confrontation of the difficulties at home or in the office.

'How do you know what level of thyroxine is normal for me?'

In the author's hospital the normal or reference range for free thyroxine (fT_4) in the blood is 10–25 picomoles per litre (pmol/l), although this will vary slightly from laboratory to laboratory. If your free T_4 is measured at 14 pmol/l, you might reasonably ask whether it should not be 20 pmol/l and, if so, whether T_4 should be given to relieve your symptoms.

The answer lies in the measurement of the pituitary hormone, TSH. By chance, the level of T_4 in the blood remains the same from day to day, month to month, and year to year in a healthy person. Any fall in the level is sensed by the pituitary gland, which increases its output of TSH in an attempt to stimulate the thyroid to produce more T_4 and return its level to its normal position.

If a normal free T_4 of 20 pmol/l fell to a value of 14 pmol/l, which is still within the reference range, the concentration of TSH in the blood would become abnormally high – an indication for considering treatment with thyroxine. If a free T_4 of 14 pmol/l is accompanied by a normal TSH concentration, this means that your free T_4 concentration is right for you and has been at that level virtually from the day you were born.

Doctors will, however, be suspicious of the combination of a low normal free T_4 of, say, 10 pmol/l and a high normal TSH of perhaps 3.2 milliunits per litre (mU/l) (normal is up to 3.5 mU/l), which may indicate that you have underlying autoimmune thyroid disease, especially if thyroid antibodies are present in your blood. Most doctors would treat you with thyroxine, not anticipating any dramatic response, but in order to prevent the onset of more severe hypothyroidism in future years.

'Why do some patients with normal blood tests feel much better when taking thyroid hormones?'

About 20 per cent of people given a dummy medicine, known as a placebo, believing it to be a real medicine, will feel better no matter what the illness is. This 'placebo effect' may last for several weeks or even months before wearing off. If you believe that you might have an underactive thyroid gland despite normal blood tests, any improvement in well-being while taking thyroxine would be the result of your relationship with a 'sympathetic' doctor who prescribes what you want. When similar patients were given either placebo or thyroxine for several weeks, not knowing which they were taking, they were unable to tell the difference. In other words, thyroxine was of no more benefit than a dummy tablet in patients who, because of symptoms such as tiredness and weight gain, thought that they had an underactive thyroid gland, although blood tests were normal.

'What is the harm in taking thyroid hormones if they make me feel better?'

There is no harm for most patients in taking a dose of thyroxine of between 50 and 75 micrograms daily. Unfortunately as the 'placebo effect' wears off you may be tempted to take higher and higher doses, which may produce the symptoms of an overactive thyroid gland. This is even more likely to occur if you are taking a combination of thyroxine and triiodothyronine, such as animal thyroid extract (for example, Armour thyroid). Although, in the short term, you may be delighted with any weight loss and apparent increase in energy, in the long term this self-induced hyperthyroidism will lead to osteoporosis and possible fracture and to an irregular heartbeat (atrial fibrillation), heart failure, stroke and even death.

'I know of some patients who are taking thyroid hormones and steroids because of symptoms like mine'

Addison's disease occurs when the adrenal glands, which sit on top of the kidneys, fail to produce enough cortisol (hydrocortisone). This occurs from time to time in patients with real hypothyroidism caused by autoimmune disease. There can, however, be no justification whatsoever for doctors prescribing steroids along with thyroid hormones for patients with symptoms of an underactive thyroid gland, but in whom thyroid blood tests have either not been taken or are normal. Steroids should never be prescribed in the belief that the adrenal glands are not working properly without adequate testing beforehand.

KEY POINTS

■ Measurements of T_4 and TSH are reliable and when taken together allow the doctor to decide when hypothyroidism is present and when it is not present

■ It is not possible to have an underactive thyroid gland with unequivocally normal levels of T_4 and TSH in the blood

■ Thyroid hormone treatment should never be started without confirmatory blood tests

Questions and answers

Do I have to change my diet?

You may have heard that iodine has something to do with the thyroid gland. Indeed iodine is an integral part of the thyroxine (T_4) and triiodothyronine (T_3) molecules. A lack of iodine in the diet may cause a goitre or even hypothyroidism. This is commonly found in people who live in mountainous areas far from the sea such as the Himalayas, but the diet in the UK contains adequate amounts of iodine and you don't need to take supplements. For the disbelievers iodised salt is available in some supermarkets. Excessive iodine intake, however, may unmask underlying thyroid disease and cause both hyperthyroidism and hypothyroidism.

Was stress responsible for making my thyroid gland overactive?

Although it is difficult to prove, most thyroid specialists are impressed by how often major life events, such as divorce or death of a close relative, appear to have taken place a few months before the onset of hyperthyroidism caused by Graves' disease. There is now evidence that stress can affect the immune system which is abnormal in Graves' disease. So the answer is probably 'yes' but there are other important factors such as heredity.

Will my new baby have thyroid trouble?

The children of mothers with Graves' disease or a previous history of Graves' disease may be born with an overactive thyroid gland. This is known as neonatal thyrotoxicosis and lasts for only a few weeks. The obstetrician and the paediatrician will be looking out for this rare complication which is readily treated.

Occasionally mothers with hypothyroidism give birth to a child with an underactive thyroid gland. Again this is usually short-lived and will be detected by the routine blood testing of all babies a few days after birth.

Will my children be affected?

Not necessarily. In fact, the risk is relatively small, although it is greater than that for children who have no family history of autoimmune disease. Nor is it always the same disease that runs in families. For example, a mother may have Graves' disease, while her daughter develops type 1 diabetes mellitus.

Could my thyroid condition explain why I did badly in my exams?

It is likely to be hyperthyroidism that affects people who are the right age to be taking exams. If it is not adequately treated, a reduced ability to concentrate will certainly lead to a substandard performance and the specialist will be happy to write to the relevant headteacher or college tutor to explain the problem.

Could thyroid disease have caused my anxiety/
depression?

The answer is almost certainly 'no', although
hyperthyroidism and hypothyroidism will make
underlying psychiatric illness worse. Unfortunately, even
when a person with hyperthyroidism is successfully
treated so that their overactive thyroid is brought under
control, their psychiatric symptoms don't disappear
altogether, although they may improve.

Will my Graves' disease recur?

If your hyperthyroidism has been effectively treated with
iodine-131, it will never return. If the hyperthyroidism
has settled after a single course of carbimazole there
is a 30 to 50 per cent chance of recurrence, usually
within 1 to 2 years of stopping the drug. Recurrent
hyperthyroidism after surgery is usually apparent within
a few weeks but may occur as long as 40 years after
apparently successful surgery.

Does it matter if I forget to take my medication?

The occasional missed tablet is not the end of the world.
Indeed symptoms of hypothyroidism caused by lack
of thyroxine are not usually felt for 2 to 3 weeks after
stopping the tablets so it would still be possible to
enjoy a 7- to 10-day holiday if you'd inadvertently left
your medication at home.

However, this is not to be recommended. Also patients
with hypothyroidism may have other autoimmune
diseases such as diabetes mellitus. Failure to take
thyroxine regularly will affect the response to insulin
and may lead to unexpected coma as a result of a low
blood sugar.

Again, missing the odd carbimazole dose will not cause significant problems but symptoms of hyperthyroidism are likely to develop if you don't take the tablets for 24 to 48 hours, especially within a few weeks of starting treatment.

I feel better when I am taking a higher dose of thyroxine than recommended by my doctor. Is this safe?
There is considerable debate about the correct dose of thyroxine. The current consensus is that enough should be given to ensure that levels of T_4 in the blood are in the upper part of the reference range or even slightly elevated, and those of TSH are in the lower part of the reference range, or even low, but not undetectable. Although, by taking excessive thyroxine, a sense of well-being, increased energy and even weight loss may be achieved in the short term, there are long-term dangers to the heart and a possibility of increasing the rate of bone thinning and therefore encouraging the development of osteoporosis.

Will tests involving radioactivity affect my fertility?
Definitely not. The amount of radioactivity involved is tiny – less than that in an X-ray – so you have absolutely no cause for concern.

Why is hypothyroidism not treated with thyroxine and triiodothyronine?
The thyroid gland manufactures both thyroxine and triiodothyronine and secretes these hormones into the bloodstream. The major source of triiodothyronine is from the conversion of the metabolically inactive thyroxine to the active triiodothyronine in the tissues and organs of the body by the action of an enzyme

that removes one atom of iodine from the thyroxine molecule. In the great majority of patients this conversion is very efficient and effective and, while taking thyroxine alone in a dose that restores thyroid blood tests to normal, they feel perfectly well. There is now some evidence to suggest that in some the conversion is not similarly efficient in all parts of the body and that is why about five per cent of patients with hypothyroidism, taking seemingly adequate doses of thyroxine, are significantly improved by taking both thyroxine and triiodothyronine. Although there have been many scientific publications that have failed to show any benefit from treatment with both hormones, most endocrinologists with busy practices are impressed by the difference that can be made in the occasional patient.

Another reason for some specialists being reluctant to agree to a trial of treatment with both thyroxine and triiodothyronine is that triiodothyronine tablets come only in a single strength of 20 micrograms; the recommended dose is 10 micrograms and the tablets are not easy to divide, even though they are scored. The usual advice is to reduce the dose of thyroxine by 25 to 50 micrograms daily and add triiodothyronine in a dose of 10 micrograms daily in the first instance. It is essential that this treatment be supervised by a specialist and that the doses are adjusted to ensure that serum TSH concentrations are normal. Although there may be uncertainty about the dangers of a low TSH while taking thyroxine alone, a low TSH while being treated with both hormones is a sign of definite overtreatment with its attendant risks of heart disease and osteoporosis and fracture.

Can treatment for Graves' disease make me fat?

No, although you will probably put back any weight you lost before your condition was diagnosed and treated.

However, there's no reason why you should end up weighing any more than you did before you started to develop Graves' disease.

My daughter was put on thyroxine at birth because she was hypothyroid. Will she have to take thyroxine forever?

Not necessarily. She will be taken off thyroxine and then given a blood test when she's around a year old to see whether she still needs it.

Is the time of day when I take my thyroxine tablets important?

Ideally, thyroxine should be taken at bedtime when there is less possibility of interference with its absorption by food or other medicines. However, the most important aspect of thyroxine treatment is that it is taken regularly and, if other times of the day are more convenient, so be it.

Should I stop smoking?

Definitely! Apart from the many health risks, such as lung cancer and heart disease, smoking reduces the effectiveness of antithyroid drugs, increases the risk of relapse at the end of treatment and may make any thyroid eye disease worse.

Glossary

This glossary explains the meaning of the most frequently used clinical and related terms connected with the diagnosis and treatment of thyroid disorders.

agranulocytosis: a rare blood disorder characterised by a severe reduction in the number of white blood cells in the circulating blood. This will leave the sufferer susceptible to a variety of bacterial infections causing symptoms such as sore throat, mouth ulcers and high fever.

antibodies: these are produced by the body's immune system as a defence mechanism against 'foreign' protein contained, for example, in bacteria. Antibodies are not normally formed against proteins that are part of the body.

autoimmune disease: antibodies are inappropriately produced which are directed against parts of the body.

For example, in most patients with hypothyroidism, antibodies are formed that participate in the destruction of the thyroid gland, whereas in Graves' disease antibodies directed against the surface of the thyroid cell stimulate it to overproduce thyroid hormones.

carbimazole: the drug most commonly used in the UK in the treatment of hyperthyroidism. It acts by interfering with the excessive production of thyroid hormones.

de Quervain's thyroiditis: a form of viral thyroiditis that can occur following a viral infection of the thyroid.

euthyroid: a term for normal thyroid function.

exophthalmos: prominence of the eyes most commonly found in patients with hyperthyroidism caused by Graves' disease. The exophthalmos may affect one or both eyes, may be apparent before the overactive thyroid gland develops and may appear for the first time after successful treatment of the hyperthyroidism.

fine needle aspiration (FNA): a test that involves passing a small needle into the thyroid gland and sucking out (aspirating) a small sample of tissue for examination under the microscope. This technique often avoids the need for surgery in patients with certain types of goitre.

genes: part of a body cell that contains the biological information of characteristics that parents pass to their children during reproduction. They control the growth and development of cells.

goitre: an enlarged thyroid gland.

Graves' disease: the name given to the most common form of hyperthyroidism. Patients often have exophthalmos, a goitre and sometimes raised red patches on the legs known as pretibial myxoedema.

Hashimoto's thyroiditis: the name given to a particular kind of goitre caused by autoimmune disease. Although the thyroid gland is enlarged, there is often evidence of hypothyroidism.

hormones: chemical messengers that alter the activity of specific target cells. They are produced in specific glands or organs and transported to their site of action in the bloodstream.

hyperthyroidism: condition resulting from an overactive thyroid gland.

hypothyroidism: condition resulting from an underactive thyroid gland.

myxoedema: this means the same as hypothyroidism, but is often used to describe patients in whom the thyroid underactivity is severe and of long standing.

postpartum thyroiditis: a transient disturbance in the balance of the thyroid gland which can occur in the first year after childbirth. There are usually no symptoms, but there may be symptoms of hyperthyroidism or hypothyroidism. Treatment is not usually necessary.

propranolol (Inderal): a drug belonging to the group known as beta blockers which alleviate some of the symptoms, for example tremor in patients with an overactive thyroid gland. Other members of the group include nadolol (Corgard) and sotalol (Sotacor).

proptosis: another word for exophthalmos.

propylthiouracil: this drug has a similar action to carbimazole. It is used if patients develop side effects to carbimazole and is prescribed to patients who are breast-feeding when hyperthyroid.

radioactive iodine (iodine-131): an isotope of iodine which is used in the investigation and treatment of hyperthyroidism.

tetany: this results from a low level of calcium in the blood with tingling in the hands, feet and around the mouth, and painful spasm of the muscles of the hands and feet.

thyroglobulin: a protein secreted by the thyroid gland. Its measurement is an important part of the follow-up of patients who have been treated for thyroid cancer. It is known as a 'tumour marker' because its presence in certain situations may indicate that the cancer has returned to other parts of the body.

thyrotoxicosis: another term for hyperthyroidism.

thyrotrophin (thyroid-stimulating hormone, TSH): a hormone secreted by the pituitary gland and responsible for controlling the output of thyroid hormones by the thyroid gland. In hypothyroidism caused by disease of the thyroid gland, TSH concentrations are elevated in the blood and in hyperthyroidism TSH concentrations are low.

thyroxine (T_4): a hormone secreted, along with triiodothyronine, by the thyroid gland. It has to be converted in the body to triiodothyronine before it is active. Thyroxine is available in tablet form for the treatment of hypothyroidism.

triiodothyronine (T_3): a hormone which, along with thyroxine, is secreted by the thyroid gland. It is responsible for controlling the metabolism of the body. Although available in tablet form, it is not usually prescribed for patients with hypothyroidism because it does not provide such good control as thyroxine.

Useful addresses

We have included the following organisations because, on preliminary investigation, they may be of use to the reader. However, we do not have first-hand experience of each organisation and so cannot guarantee the organisation's integrity. The reader must therefore exercise his or her own discretion and judgement when making further enquiries.

Benefit Enquiry Line
Tel: 0800 882200 (Mon–Fri 8am–6pm)
Textphone: 0800 243355
Website: www.gov.uk/benefit-enquiry-line

Government agency giving information and advice on sickness and disability benefits for people with disabilities and their carers.

British Thyroid Foundation X
2nd Floor, 3 Devonshire Place
Harrogate, North Yorkshire HG1 4AA

Tel: 01423 709707 or 01423 709448
Website: www.btf-thyroid.org

Provides support and information to sufferers of thyroid disorders, promotes a greater awareness of these disorders among the general public and medical profession, helps set up regional support groups and raises funds for research.

National Institute for Health and Clinical Excellence (NICE)

1st Floor, 10 Spring Gardens
London SW1A 2BU
Tel: 0845 003 7784
Website: www.nice.org.uk

Provides national guidance on the promotion of good health and treatment of ill-health. Patient information leaflets are available for each piece of guidance issued.

NHS Direct

Tel: 0845 4647 (24 hours, 365 days a year)
Website: www.nhsdirect.nhs.uk

Offers confidential health-care advice, information and referral service. A good first port of call for any health advice.

NHS Smoking Helpline

Freephone: 0800 022 4332 (Mon–Fri 9am–8pm, Sat & Sun 11am–4pm)
Website: http://smokefree.nhs.uk

Have advice, help and encouragement on giving up smoking. Specialist advisers available to offer ongoing support to those who genuinely are trying to give up smoking. Can refer to local branches.

Patients' Association
PO Box 935
Harrow, Middlesex HA1 3YJ
Helpline: 0845 608 4455
Tel: 020 8423 9111
Website: www.patients-association.com

Provides advice on patients' rights, leaflets and a directory of self-help groups.

Quit (Smoking Quitlines)
20 Curtain Road
London EC2A 3NF
Helpline: 0800 002200 (Mon–Fri 9am–8pm, Sat, Sun 10am–4pm)
Tel: 020 7539 1700
Website: www.quit.org.uk

Offers individual advice on giving up smoking in English and Asian languages. Talks to schools on smoking and pregnancy and can refer to local support groups. Runs training courses for professionals.

Thyroid Eye Disease Charitable Trust (TEDct)
PO Box 1928
Bristol BS37 0AX
Tel: 0844 800 8133
Website: www.tedct.co.uk

Offers information, care and support to those affected by thyroid eye disease via UK-wide support groups and telephone helplines. Raises awareness of the condition among the medical profession and general public, and fund raises for research.

Useful websites

BBC
www.bbc.co.uk/health
A helpful website: easy to navigate and offers lots of useful advice and information. Also contains links to other related topics.

Healthtalkonline
www.healthtalkonline.org
Website of the DIPEx charity.

NHS choices
www.nhs.uk/conditions
Government's patient information portal.

Patient UK
www.patient.co.uk
Patient care website.

The internet as a source of further information

After reading this book, you may feel that you would like further information on the subject. The internet is of course an excellent place to look and there are many websites with useful information about medical disorders, related charities and support groups.

It should always be remembered, however, that the internet is unregulated and anyone is free to set up a website and add information to it. Many websites offer impartial advice and information that has been compiled and checked by qualified medical professionals. Some, on the other hand, are run by commercial organisations with the purpose of promoting their own products. Others still are run by pressure groups, some of which will provide carefully assessed and accurate information whereas others may be suggesting medications or treatments that are not supported by the medical and scientific community.

Unless you know the address of the website you want to visit – for example, www.familydoctor.co.uk – you may find the following guidelines useful when searching the internet for information.

Search engines and other searchable sites

Google (www.google.co.uk) is the most popular search engine used in the UK, followed by Yahoo! (http://uk.yahoo.com) and MSN (www.msn.co.uk). Also popular are the search engines provided by Internet Service Providers such as TalkTalk and other sites such as the BBC site (www.bbc.co.uk).

In addition to the search engines that index the whole web, there are also medical sites with search facilities, which act almost like mini-search engines, but cover only medical topics or even a particular area of medicine. Again, it is wise to look at who is responsible for compiling the information offered to ensure that it is impartial and medically accurate. The NHS Direct site (www.nhsdirect.nhs.uk) is an example of a searchable medical site.

Links to many British medical charities can be found at the Association of Medical Research Charities' website (www.amrc.org.uk) and at Charity Choice (www.charitychoice.co.uk).

Search phrases

Be specific when entering a search phrase. Searching for information on 'cancer' will return results for many different types of cancer as well as on cancer in general. You may even find sites offering astrological information. More useful results will be returned by using search phrases such as 'lung cancer' and 'treatments for lung cancer'. Both Google and Yahoo! offer an advanced search option that includes the ability to search for the exact phrase; enclosing the search phrase in quotes, that is, 'treatments for lung cancer', will have the same effect. Limiting a search to an exact phrase reduces the number of results returned but it is best to refine a search to an exact match only if you are not getting useful results with a normal search. Adding 'UK' to your search term will bring up mainly British sites, so a good phrase might be 'lung cancer' UK (don't include UK within the quotes).

Always remember the internet is international and unregulated. It holds a wealth of valuable information but individual sites may be biased, out of date or just plain wrong. Family Doctor Publications accepts no responsibility for the content of links published in this series.

Index

Your pages

We have included the following pages because they may help you manage your illness or condition and its treatment.

Before an appointment with a health professional, it can be useful to write down a short list of questions of things that you do not understand, so that you can make sure that you do not forget anything.

Some of the sections may not be relevant to your circumstances.

We are always pleased to receive constructive criticism or suggestions about how to improve the books. You can contact us at:

Email: familydoctor@btinternet.com
Letter: Family Doctor Publications
         PO Box 4664
         Poole
         BH15 1NN

Thank you

Health-care contact details

Name:

Job title:

Place of work:

Tel:

Name:

Job title:

Place of work:

Tel:

Name:

Job title:

Place of work:

Tel:

Name:

Job title:

Place of work:

Tel:

Significant past health events – illnesses/ operations/investigations/treatments

Event	Month	Year	Age (at time)

Appointments for health care

Name:

Place:

Date:

Time:

Tel:

Name:

Place:

Date:

Time:

Tel:

Name:

Place:

Date:

Time:

Tel:

Name:

Place:

Date:

Time:

Tel:

Appointments for health care

Name:

Place:

Date:

Time:

Tel:

Name:

Place:

Date:

Time:

Tel:

Name:

Place:

Date:

Time:

Tel:

Name:

Place:

Date:

Time:

Tel:

Current medication(s) prescribed by your doctor

Medicine name:

Purpose:

Frequency & dose:

Start date:

End date:

Medicine name:

Purpose:

Frequency & dose:

Start date:

End date:

Medicine name:

Purpose:

Frequency & dose:

Start date:

End date:

Medicine name:

Purpose:

Frequency & dose:

Start date:

End date:

Other medicines/supplements you are taking, not prescribed by your doctor

Medicine/treatment:

Purpose:

Frequency & dose:

Start date:

End date:

Medicine/treatment:

Purpose:

Frequency & dose:

Start date:

End date:

Medicine/treatment:

Purpose:

Frequency & dose:

Start date:

End date:

Medicine/treatment:

Purpose:

Frequency & dose:

Start date:

End date:

Questions to ask at appointments
(Note: do bear in mind that doctors work under great time pressure, so long lists may not be helpful for either of you)

Questions to ask at appointments
(Note: do bear in mind that doctors work under great time
pressure, so long lists may not be helpful for either of you)

Notes